SOMETHING FEELS OFF

Thriving in Life & Business Beyond a Mental Health Crisis

By Laura Watkins, MBA

Edited by Becky J. Sasso

Invisible Ink

invisibleinkbooks.com

Paperback ISBN 979-8-9987171-0-9

eBook ISBN 979-8-9987171-1-6

Copyright © 2025 by Laura Watkins

All rights reserved.

This memoir is a reflection of the author's personal experiences and is presented as remembered to the best of their ability. Some names, identifying details, and locations have been changed or altered for privacy and storytelling purposes. While every effort has been made to remain true to the spirit of the events, certain scenes have been reconstructed or adapted to enhance narrative flow and readability.

Canva pro images have been altered from their original form and are authorized under article 5, section 6 of Canva's Content License agreement.

No part of this book may be reproduced in any form or by any electronic or mechanical means, including information storage and retrieval systems, without written permission from the author, except for the use of brief quotations in a book review.

Cover & interior by Becky J. Sasso, Invisible Ink Books

To my husband, Mike—my greatest love, protector, and supporter. I know you would have moved mountains if you thought it would make me well again. Thank you for always believing in me and my audacious pursuits.

Contents

Content Warning	vii
Introduction	ix
1. The Silent Battle	1
2. Wide Open Spaces	7
3. Corporate America Dropout	15
4. Fake It Til You Make It	21
5. Maybe You Should Pray More	26
6. Beach Weekend	31
7. California Rocket Fuel	39
8. The Lights Come Back On	53
9. Coming Out of the Mental Illness Closet	68
10. The Awakening	83
11. Let's Change the Conversation	98
Laura's Self-Care Toolkit	109
Resources	111
Acknowledgments	113
About the Author	117

Content Warning

This book contains discussions of mental health challenges, including treatment-resistant depression and suicidal ideation. These topics may be distressing or triggering for some readers. Please prioritize your emotional well-being as you read and take breaks or seek support if needed.

If you or someone you know is struggling, you are not alone. Help is available.

For immediate support in the United States, contact the Suicide & Crisis Lifeline by dialing 988—available 24/7, free, and confidential.

Introduction

Each year, one in five adults in the United States is diagnosed with a mental illness (NAMI). Behind that statistic are millions of stories—stories of heartbreak, perseverance, and, sometimes, transformation. *Something Feels Off* is one of those rare and remarkable stories.

Laura Watkins is nothing short of extraordinary. A badass businesswoman, she earned her MBA, became a trained cosmetologist, and built a thriving Aveda salon in her hometown of Louisville with a clear vision and unmatched drive. She's also the fiercely loving wife of a retired Army husband and devoted mother of two daughters. But like so many high-functioning women, Laura carried an invisible weight—one that too often goes unseen behind success, service, and a smile.

What makes Laura so inspiring isn't just what she's achieved; it's who she has become through pain. I think the wisest and most empathetic people are those who have suffered deeply and grown anyway—and Laura is no exception. She has not only battled the darkness of major depressive disorder, but she has emerged from it with the courage to speak her truth and advocate for others. As a business owner, she is working to transform the culture of the salon industry by doing what few leaders are brave enough to do: priori-

Introduction

tize mental health in the workplace. Her commitment to creating a salon environment that supports emotional wellness is groundbreaking—and deeply needed.

This book chronicles the incredible tenacity Laura showed in searching for answers, even when traditional medicine and many of the standard treatments failed her. Even when she was exhausted and beaten down, she refused to give up on herself. And that resilience? It's the lifeblood of this memoir. It takes a rare kind of person to turn suffering into service—to use personal pain as a platform for hope. Laura has done exactly that.

After nearly two decades editing books, I've worked on close to 100 manuscripts. I may forget the finer details or a turn of phrase, but I never forget how a project makes me *feel*. This book injected me with hope. Working with Laura made me feel seen in my own mental health journey, and reminded me that the highest honor is to help inspire the healing of another. That privilege is afforded to very few—and Laura wears it with grace.

Something Feels Off is not just a story about mental illness—it's a story about rediscovering your power, finding purpose, and rising again. It is also the perfect first book to publish under my brand new, woman-owned publishing imprint, created to uplift bold female voices of transformation. Laura's journey is raw, real, and deeply moving—and I can't wait for you to experience it.

Becky J. Sasso

Founder, Invisible Ink Books

Chapter 1

The Silent Battle

"God bless you." said Dr. Stewart as my mom and I left his office.

What an odd thing to say to me right now, I thought.

I could barely put one foot in front of the other since finishing yet another treatment that didn't work for my crippling depression. His words angered me because they sounded so simple, definitive, and dismissive. He was sending me out the door to another doctor who may or may not be able to help me. That felt even more hopeless. I didn't have the energy for another round of treatment that wasn't guaranteed to work. I had tried multiple unsuccessful medications already and this was the third psychiatrist, a supposed expert in treating Major Depressive Disorder, who had failed me. This shit had been going on for four years now and I was getting so tired of fighting. I woke up every day exhausted and in so much emotional pain that I could not fathom going on like this much longer.

The relentless attacks of negative self-talk that I combatted every day had taken an immense toll on me, my family, my staff, and anyone who loved and cared about me. My brain told me I had asked too much of them. That they had to be sick of me being unwell. I convinced myself that they were tired of watching me cry again. No matter how hard I tried to explain how I was feeling and make them understand the hell I lived in every day inside my head, I was unsuccessful.

Even now it's hard to find the words to describe what that level of mental anguish actually feels like. My thoughts were a continuous loop that told me, I'm not worth all of this. I'm a terrible example for my children. I'm a terrible wife for putting my husband through this for so long. I'm a grown woman but I need my mom, dad, and sister to take turns coming over every day to lead me through the most basic tasks. Things like deciding what to fix for dinner or throwing in a load of laundry were just too overwhelming to think about doing alone.

My parents haven't had to tell me to take a shower or bathe myself for at least 40 years but just last week my mom asked me, "When was the last time you took a shower?" She meant it in the most loving, non-judgmental way but the sickness in my brain told me over and over how disgusting I was and what a disappointment I must be to her.

This time my depression was darker than it had ever been, scary dark. Scarier than any scene in a horror movie because the monster who was trying to kill me was an invisible, persistent part of myself. A voice inside of me that no one else could hear telling me over and over again how pointless it was to be alive and all of the ways in which I had failed. In the last four years, I had brief periods of relief from my depression. Each reprieve, I would be so hopeful that maybe this time was different. I would go back to work and be able to live independently for a while and enjoy moments with my girls and husband.

Inevitably, the medication would stop working.

I would deny, deny, deny it when my husband would ask, "It's happening again, isn't it?" after he'd been through this cycle with me repeatedly and knew what to look for.

"No!" I would insist it wasn't happening again for a few days, or even a week, before I couldn't fake it anymore. I would feel like a complete failure because I couldn't stay well.

No amount of exercise, journaling, gratitude, or intentional breathing could stop it from happening. Each period of depression felt like a personal failure to thrive. I would spiral down farther than the time before, to a place I could not climb out of on my own. I would go months without being able to work or make decisions of any kind.

Luckily, I have an incredible manager on my team at Pure Salon Spa, the small Aveda salon I own in Louisville, Kentucky. She kept things going during my many absences and allowed me to keep my business open.

This time, I started to consider how I would end the pain on my own if this went on much longer. I even got so far as to decide how I would kill myself if it came to that. Due to my complete lack of a pain tolerance, I decided on what I considered the most peaceful way to do it without leaving a mess for someone else to clean up. This would be to pull my car into the garage, close the door, leave the car running, and fall into a deep sleep I wouldn't wake up from.

I never thought in my wildest dreams I would get to a point where I would actually consider suicide. I used to think that was so selfish and wonder how anyone could do it. I get it now. In such an intimate way that I wish like hell that I didn't.

When you get to the stage of mental illness that you want to kill yourself, you begin to stop considering the consequences of an act like that. You push things like who would find you or how much pain you would cause the people who love you to the back of your mind. They seem like small prices to pay for the absolute relief you could give yourself by not being alive. For not having to feel the anguish anymore or listen to the shameful things your brain repeats that only stop when you are asleep. Just deciding how you would kill yourself provides a little relief, especially in my case when nothing else I had tried was working.

That day, as my mom and I sat on the couch in Dr. Stewart's office, I explained to him how the Ketamine infusions I'd been receiving hadn't left me feeling any less depressed. For the last two weeks, I came to his office every other day to receive an intravenous infusion of Ketamine. Ketamine is a drug that induces a trance-like state that provides pain relief, sedation, and amnesia. Commonly-used as anesthesia in veterinary medicine, Ketamine was used extensively as surgical anesthesia in the Vietnam War (Wikipedia). Ketamine can also be bought "on the streets" referred to as Special K or simply "K" and is widely used recreationally for its hallucinogenic and dissociative effects. Most recently, Ketamine has gained notoriety as a treatment for depression. (Grinspoon)

Although it scared me to try that type of drug as part of my treatment, I was desperate. So far, I hadn't found a combination of medications that kept me well. Plus, it didn't sound as invasive to me as Electroconvulsive therapy (ECT), so I gave it a try. ECT is a treatment for various mental illnesses that involves going to the hospital, being put to sleep, and a psychiatrist placing electrodes on each of your temples. The electrodes send electrical current coursing through your brain to induce a mild seizure. (Mayo) This process serves as a reset and, after a series of treatments, can improve symptoms of mental illness. This treatment option was suggested to me by a psychiatrist I saw prior to Dr. Stewart. At the time, the procedure seemed much too scary and the risks far too great.

Each Ketamine infusion began with a nurse starting an IV on me. After a short amount of time, the slow drip of Ketamine into my veins made me feel like I was flying. The treatment gave me such a relief from all my mental anguish, until I was unhooked and the drug wasn't coursing through my veins, and the depression remained. After my last Ketamine infusion, we met with the practice's psychiatrist to give him an update and see what next steps he suggested. After some other pleasantries that I don't remember, Dr. Stewart mentioned a colleague who spent most of his career performing ECT for patients with treatment resistant major depressive disorder. There it was again, two years later, another doctor was suggesting I look into ECT and this time I was listening. What did I have to lose? If ECT did work, maybe it could be the miracle I was looking for. If it didn't work, I already had a plan on how to end the pain myself.

I had decided this would be the last ditch effort in this fight for me. Any of the fears I had before had been diminished with the years I had spent battling this terrible illness. They seemed like a small price to pay to be able to live normally again.

Fine. I thought. *I'll try your damn ECT.*

I set up an appointment to meet with Dr. Stewart's colleague, Dr. Burke, at The Brook Hospital to discuss my medical history and see what he had to say. My husband, Mike, and I went to the appointment together and gave Dr. Burke the details of my mental health journey. We told him the names of all of the medications I'd tried and the treatments I'd done like Transcranial Magnetic Stimulation (TMS) and Ketamine Infusions all in an effort to snap me out of my depression. We talked about all of the stressful times in my life up to this point, including my parent's divorce, army deployments that took Mike away for months at a time, several moves with the military, and starting a business. Among other things that I still didn't consider "bad enough" to cause a case of depression as severe as mine.

"Can you think of anything else that I may need to know about to treat you?" Dr. Burke asked when we were finished. Mike and I looked at each other and shook our heads.

"I think you'd be a great candidate for ECT." he said and proceeded to share what the preparation required. I would have to get approved by my primary care physician, ensuring that I was in good physical condition to do this type of treatment. This really boiled down to a series of blood tests and an EKG to make sure my heart could withstand the treatment. I got everything done and scheduled a series of six ECT treatments to start a couple of weeks before Thanksgiving in 2019.

All I had left to do was to have the results from my primary care physician sent over to Dr. Burke's office, so they could get everything approved by my insurance. Despite many attempts and reminders to both offices, their sense of urgency was never in line with mine, and the paperwork hadn't yet made it to Dr. Burke. It was Thursday morning and my first treatment was scheduled for the following Monday.

It was my Dad's day to babysit me and he decided to take me and just show up at the doctor's office to demand my paperwork be sent. Had I been well, I could have asserted myself in a way that would have gotten this done. In my depressed state, I wasn't capable of executing the most basic things, much less having the confidence or fortitude to deal with the doctor's office and insist on the result I needed.

We walked up to the counter and the lady barely looked at me when she asked dully, "What's the name?"

I wanted to scream. *MY FUCKING NAME IS LAURA WATKINS AND YOU SHOULD KNOW WHO I AM BECAUSE I'VE BEEN CALLING THIS OFFICE EVERY DAMN DAY ASKING FOR MY RECORDS TO BE SENT TO DOCTOR BURKE, WHO IS GOING TO SAVE MY LIFE, BUT YOU ASSHOLES HAVEN'T BEEN ABLE TO GET IT DONE YET. SO, I'M NOT GOING TO LEAVE UNTIL YOU DO IT RIGHT NOW!*

Instead, I looked weakly over at my Dad, my eyes pleading with him to say it for me.

Chapter 2

Wide Open Spaces

I was born into a loving family, the oldest of two girls, and grew up in the suburbs just south of Louisville, Kentucky. My parents were both educated and nurturing, providing a secure household for us to grow up in. My mom stayed home with us until I was in high school, while my dad was a businessman who worked in sales. We sat down to a home-cooked meal together every night and were taught to be polite, respectful, and to appreciate how fortunate we were.

When I was in high school, my parents built a house with a horseshoe driveway out front. I thought that was pretty freaking cool. We moved to what was considered at the time a bougie neighborhood where the wealthier residents of the county lived. We weren't rich by any means, but we had nice things. We took enjoyable vacations, lived in a modern home, and were encouraged to excel in school so we could have similar opportunities when we grew up.

My parents had high expectations for us—something that was both annoying as a teenager and, in hindsight, the greatest gift they could have given us. I realize now that holding me accountable, expecting me to make the honor roll, and insisting I call to order the pizza instead of doing it for me were lessons designed to prepare me for what life would throw my way. They didn't give in very often, and my mom had a particular look she would give us when we crossed the line—a look we jokingly called the "laser look." It meant we'd better stop, or else.

My parents had high expectations for myself and my sister, but not everybody did. During high school, I learned what it felt like to be treated differently because I was female.

My political science teacher was a tall man, likely in his 40s at the time, with thinning hair. He was also a baseball coach and, at some point, had been hit by a ball that jammed his pointer finger into a permanent bend. That bent finger was all I could see when he pointed to call on someone in class. One day, as we sat in class, he pointed that finger at one of my male classmates, who gave an incorrect answer.

"I guess we have to ask a girl now," he said in a snarky tone.

Another time, he addressed the class randomly, saying, "Nothing good comes out of Bullitt County. Most of you will end up flipping burgers or barefoot and pregnant."

The more he made these kinds of comments, the more furious I became. It seemed so unfair for him to make such assumptions about all the girls, and I would usually be seething by the time class ended. Every day, I had to sit and listen to this man belittle the girls in the class while acting as though the boys could do no wrong. I wondered if he trying, in some misguided way, to motivate us to have higher expectations for ourselves?

I considered reporting him to the school administrators but changed my mind the day my principal casually asked if I was going to college to get my "MRS degree." WTF? This small-town, backward manner of thinking made my blood boil. At the time, however, I hadn't yet found my voice. I was still trying to be the polite, respectful young woman I was "supposed" to be.

I was brought up in the "suck it up" generation, by parents who subscribed to that mentality. It was okay to cry and talk about our feelings, but once the crying and talking were done, you were expected to soldier on. This approach served me well in many scenarios. Until it didn't. Part of the human experience is feeling sadness, disappointment, heartbreak, fear, stress, or nervousness. Typically, with the right tools and examples to follow, people can work through it. Resilience is something my family prides itself on, and it gave me strength to achieve accomplishments I'm still proud of.

For example, I was in the marching band during high school and earned the position of field commander. That's the person who leads everyone onto the football field and conducts the music while the band moves in formation. That was me. I had a fancy uniform, performed a special salute at the start of each performance, and presented the entire band as we hit the crescendo of a song and marched forward on the 50-yard line toward the crowd. I even brought home the first trophy my high school ever won for best field commander in our category at the Kentucky State Fair band competition during my senior year. This wasn't my first experience as a field commander; I also held the role in middle school, despite my band teacher initially telling me I was too short. I proved her wrong during auditions, showing her that height had nothing to do with talent or passion. So, yeah—don't tell me I can't do something because that only fuels my desire to prove otherwise.

When it came to plans after high school, I didn't realize there was a choice about whether I would attend college or not. For me, the only question was *where* I would go. I graduated from the University of Louisville in 1995 with a degree in Marketing. Those four and a half years of college were some of the best days of my life. I graduated with no debt, lifelong friendships from my sorority, and a readiness to launch my career as an eager, independent young woman determined to set the world on fire. I went on to earn my Master's in Business Administration in 2000. My 20s were a blast, filled with exciting experiences in corporate marketing, but I always knew I wanted to start my own business someday, just as my dad had done while I was in high school.

However, during these years, my parents' marriage began to unravel. They eventually divorced when I was 21, marking my first experience with trauma. Even now, I hesitate to label their divorce as trauma because it didn't fit my then-perception of what trauma was "supposed" to be. I associated trauma with really serious stuff like like sexual assault, physical abuse, kidnapping, or catastrophic accidents that left you paralyzed.

While those things are definitely traumatic, my parents' divorce seemed insignificant by comparison. Yet, at 21, when your parents decide to separate after 23 years of marriage—and you've never even seen them fight—it feels deeply traumatizing. I felt like my life had been a charade up until that point. My parents had always presented a united front, supporting me through breakups, family losses, failures, and disappointments.

They also celebrated my milestones like prom and graduation together. Even their discipline was a team effort, grounding me for coming home late or lying about where I'd been. They gave me the impression that we were a "special" family, immune to the misfortunes that befell others, like divorce. We ate dinner together every night, went to church every weekend, and enjoyed fellowship with close family friends. Divorce was something that happened to other families—not ours.

When it did happen, my entire world seemed to crumble. Suddenly, I was left to figure out how to move forward in life with my parents no longer together. It was a confusing time, made worse by well-meaning but misguided comments like, "Oh, it must have been easier since you were already an adult and out of the house. At least you didn't have to be shuffled back and forth as a kid."

I'd think to myself, *Maybe that's true.* But those people didn't consider how devastating it was to no longer have the comfort of returning from college to my family home. Instead, I had to navigate two separate, unfamiliar homes. For me, the phrase "there's no place like home" no longer applied. So no, it wasn't easier. Divorce sucks no matter how old you are when it happens.

During my parents' divorce, I was introduced to talk therapy. It seemed like such a big deal at the time to be seeing a therapist. I didn't know anyone personally who saw a therapist and any impressions I had about therapy were from movies or TV shows. I assumed there had to be something pretty serious going on to get a therapist involved.

I don't remember mental health being a topic of discussion during my childhood. As far as I knew, we didn't have anyone close to us who struggled with it. I don't recall talking about mental health with high school friends or hearing anyone mention they were dealing with anxiety or depression. Back then, we'd joke about being sent to a mental institution if we were stressed or having a "crazy" day. The old, abandoned mental hospital in Louisville had a reputation as a spooky place teenagers went on Halloween. The words "crazy," "scary," and "torture" were what I associated with mental institutions—and anyone who spent time in one had to be, in my uninformed view, batshit crazy. Those were my perceptions, no matter how wrong they were.

Now I believe that everyone should have a therapist. I don't think twice about setting up time with mine when I'm facing a challenge or a difficult season in life. Checking in on your mental health should be as common as getting a routine checkup with your primary care physician. Unfortunately, matters of the brain are not yet prioritized like other physical ailments.

Unbeknownst to me, my parents had been in therapy with a counselor named Peter for several years prior to divorcing. We each had the opportunity to talk to Peter about how we felt in the aftermath of the divorce. I leaned into this process and gained a lot from it. Looking back, I realize that exposure to therapy during this period was an unrecognized gift of my parents' divorce. It became an essential tool in my later battles with depression and has a permanent place in my self-care routine.

The confusion and anger I felt during my parents' divorce fueled a reckless phase of drinking and making poor choices with guys. Let's just say, I'm glad there weren't iPhones or social media back then. At the same time, my anger ignited a fierce independence and a "girl power" mantra that remains an essential part of who I am today. I excelled at most things I set my sights on and was never afraid to outwork anyone to achieve my goals. This earned me the reputation of being an "overachiever," but I didn't care. I carried that same determination through college, where I maintained grades high enough to be accepted into business school while juggling a busy social life and navigating my parents' divorce.

I met lifelong friends in college, and through those relationships, I began to see how different everyone's upbringing was. Not better or worse, just different. In my junior year of college, I met Robin, who is still a close friend to this day. We occasionally spent time at her parents' house. Her dad worked a lot and wasn't home much when I visited, but her mom, Julie, was usually there. Most of my interactions with Julie happened while Robin and I chatted with her in bed. The first time Robin invited me to her house, she explained that Julie suffered from depression, which was why she was often in bed during the day. I found it odd at first, as I had never known anyone with depression—let alone someone who stayed in bed all day because of it. But Robin was a close friend, and after the initial surprise, it became normal.

The more I got to know Julie, the more I saw her humor and warmth. On good days, she lit up the room, loved to laugh, and even joined us for nights out dancing and listening to live music. She was creative, fun, and full of life. Yet, on other days, she'd barely be able to stay awake. It was confusing to see someone so vibrant reduced to such a low state. I still didn't fully understand mental illness or how it could take away the simple things most of us take for granted. Back then, I still had the luxury of judgement. There was part of me that couldn't understand Julie for not being able to "snap out of it." I wondered why she couldn't do a better job of being there for her family or get a job, like all of the other adults I knew.

Unfortunately Julie passed away several years ago. I'd give anything to be able to talk to her one more time and let her know I understand now. I know what she was going through and how hard she was fighting. I would tell her that both things can be true—we can be amazing women *and* somebody battling depression. The depression doesn't define us. During those formative years, I began to find my voice and confidence through my sorority experiences and leadership roles, embracing the sentiment: *I am woman, hear me roar!* I was sassy, fun, and often the instigator of mischief among my friends. Those were some of the best years of my life.

After college, I started working in the marketing department of an emerging communications company. It was a crash course in navigating corporate structures, and I was fortunate to travel and gain exposure to business situations I wasn't remotely prepared for—but I was too naïve to realize it. On one trip, I visited Southern California for the first time. I immediately fell in love with the weather and culture, so different from Kentucky. My company had an office in Irvine, California, and I began dreaming of transferring there to live by the beach. Around that same time, the Dixie Chicks released "Wide Open Spaces," a song about striking out to find a dream and a life of your own. That song became my anthem and solidified my California dream. I confidently told HR and my parents I was moving within the year and started planning.

Before the move, I visited a college friend, Joann, in Savannah, Georgia. She was living with her fiancé, who was stationed there with the Army. She invited me to stay during the big St. Patrick's Day celebration, and I was excited to experience that and see her new life. During the visit, I met Mike—her fiancé's brother. The moment Mike walked in, wearing camouflage fatigues, black boots, and that hat, my heart skipped a beat. Over the weekend, we spent a lot of time together, laughing and flirting, although he had a girlfriend and I was only a couple of months away from moving to California. Despite the obvious spark between us, my plans wouldn't be derailed by some guy—not even him. Plus, he was taken and I had an aversion to military guys—or so I thought.

Two months later, I packed up my white, five-speed Mitsubishi Eclipse and hit the road to California with a friend. I was ready to leave everything I'd ever known behind for a new adventure out West.

Chapter 3

Corporate America Dropout

It would be another year before Mike and I admitted our true feelings for each other and decided to try a long-distance relationship. By that time, I was a year into living my California dream, while he was still stationed in Savannah, Georgia. We were about as far apart as two people could get in the US, but we made it work. I would fly out to visit him, he did the same, and occasionally we'd meet back in Louisville, where his brother and Joann, now married, had moved. For more than two years, we continued this way before deciding to take the next step in our relationship.

During that time, Mike received his first orders to deploy to Kosovo for six months. Though we rarely saw each other in person, the thought of him being even farther away, in a foreign country with limited access to communication, was devastating. I had never experienced anything like it before. Yet, I knew this would happen again if I chose to stay with him long-term as he continued his Army career. True to form, I confidently pushed through it because I believed our relationship was worth it.

While Mike was deployed, I missed him terribly. Communication options back then were limited to letters, occasional emails, and sporadic phone calls, usually only every week or two. I pounced on the phone whenever it rang, hoping desperately it was him. Most of his calls came in the middle of the night because of the time difference, but I didn't care. One particularly memorable call came at 2 am on September 11, 2001. Mike called to wish me a happy birthday and tell me he loved me. I hung up feeling warm, loved, and grateful. A couple of hours later, I was jolted awake by my roommate yelling from the living room.

"Oh my God!" she screamed. "They just hit the second tower!"

I stumbled out of bed, confused, and found her watching the news. We stood frozen as we watched the horror unfold. Our country was under attack by terrorists. My mind raced: *What does this mean? What should we do? Will there be more attacks? Are big cities like Los Angeles next? Is my family in Kentucky safe?* My thoughts turned to Mike. *Is he safe? Are US troops being attacked, too?*

I had just talked to him hours earlier, and now I wouldn't hear from him again for at least a week. The fear and uncertainty were overwhelming. Fortunately, no additional cities were attacked, I reached my family quickly, and I heard from Mike a few days later. Though the days following 9/11 were unsettling and full of uncertainty, I focused on counting down the days until Mike returned from Kosovo.

One night, a phone call from Mike changed everything. From a makeshift bathroom in the desert—one of the few places he could find privacy—he asked, "What would you think about moving with me to Richmond, Virginia, later this year while I attend my captain's course?"

I laughed. "You're asking me to leave my job and the beach and move across the country, to a place you'll only be for eight months before moving again?"

"Yes." he replied, "My parents love you. And my friends don't think you're a bitch, so why not?"

That was classic Mike—endearingly blunt and funny. Secretly, I had been longing to be closer to him, though my career-minded independent streak would never let me admit it.

"I'll tell you what," I said. "I'll make one move as your girlfriend, but if we're not engaged by the end of these eight months in Virginia, I'm out."

Richmond was a blast. We moved into a one-bedroom apartment and enjoyed getting to know each other better while I started adapting to military life. By month seven, I was nervous—still no ring, and I was already planning my next move. But Mike surprised me with a proposal. Soon we were heading to his next assignment at Ft. Campbell, home of the 101st Airborne Division, and a new house in Clarksville, Tennessee.

Clarksville was a hard adjustment. It was remote—a stark contrast to life in Richmond or Southern California. Only a few months after settling in, Mike came home with crushing news: "My unit is being deployed to Iraq in about a month."

The announcement hit me like a gut punch, though I knew it was inevitable. Ft. Campbell was one of the most combat-ready posts in the country and rumors of Saddam Hussein's weapons of mass destruction were all over the news. I knew when I chose a soldier as my life partner there would be sacrifices and periods of time alone, but this was too soon. Although it wasn't how I had imagined my wedding, we decided to marry in a small ceremony surrounded by family and friends before he left. Before I knew it, I was alone in a new house, in a new world as a military spouse, with little knowledge of what that role entailed. I was terrified.

Mike's first deployment lasted a few months, but it wasn't his last. While he was gone, the US military invaded Iraq, which made this experience different than when he was in Kosovo on a humanitarian deployment. This was the first stage of the Iraq war and everyone's fears were escalating. The news stories included speeches by President Bush, stories about combat operations, airstrikes, protests, and the capture of Saddam Hussein.

As Mike's deployment progressed, the war on terror was announced and more stories were told about US troops being injured, captured or killed in combat. I attended support groups (FRG- Family Readiness Groups) for the families of deployed soldiers, even though, in many ways, I felt like an outsider. Some of the women had years of experience with military life. Many of them had chosen to forgo careers of their own to devote themselves to the careers of their husbands. That was a choice I respected, but one I knew I could never make.

I loved Mike and was proud of his service, but I had my own goals. I felt the other wives viewed me as less committed for not making the same choices as they had. I struggled to figure out where I fit among them, until I finally met Melinda. She was the wife of one of the guys in Mike's unit. She became my ride-or-die friend and is probably the main reason I survived that first deployment experience. Luckily, the company I worked for in Richmond agreed to let me work remotely after we moved. Attending to my work responsibilities gave me purpose and allowed me to stay in touch with a career-oriented mindset while navigating my new reality as a military spouse.

During Mike's second deployment, I had a life-changing conversation with a co-worker. We were venting about our corporate jobs when she asked me a question that changed the trajectory of my career, and life for that matter: "If money and location didn't matter, what would you do with your career?"

Without hesitation, I replied, "I'd quit my job, go to cosmetology school, and open an Aveda salon."

She exclaimed, "You should do it! You're always talking about Aveda and beauty—you'd be amazing!"

The idea planted a seed I couldn't ignore. When Mike returned, I told him my decision. "I'm quitting my job, going to cosmetology school, and opening an Aveda salon."

He blinked. "You do realize you have an MBA, right? And now you want to go to *beauty school?*"

"Yes," I said firmly.

To his credit, Mike supported my decision, and has continued to do this throughout our marriage. He knew I was determined once my mind was made up. At 30 years old, I left a decade-long career in corporate marketing and enrolled at New Directions Hair Academy in Nashville, a 45-minute commute from my home in Clarksville. The transition was a culture shock—I was one of the oldest students and among the few married ones. Pregnant with my first daughter, Julia, I graduated with my cosmetology license two months before she was born.

Life became even more challenging after Julia's arrival in July of 2005. Mike deployed in November to Iraq for a year, leaving me to navigate both new motherhood and career alone. I struggled with "mom guilt," juggling daycare and work while missing Mike and worrying for his safety.

This deployment was much more intense than the others. Mike had been assigned to a different unit and Melinda moved to her husband's next assignment at a new location. I was thrown into a new group of wives I didn't know. As Mike was now a Captain, I had gained the rank of Captain's wife, which came with a whole new set of expectations among the other wives in his unit.

I was worn thin and spent much of my time battling my own thoughts. I was consumed with fears about how I was doing as a mom, wife, and hairstylist. Not to mention, worrying whether my husband would come home unscathed from his latest experience in Iraq. Anxiety crept in and wouldn't leave. It hung around me like a cloud and finally became bad enough that I made a doctors appointment, culminating in my first prescription for Lexapro. I believe it helped me regain my control and perspective, but I felt embarrassed and weak for needing medication to cope with my life.

I had support from my family, who would come for visits and

help me with Julia while I worked. Still, most of my time was spent alone with Julia or gathering with other wives to vent our frustrations and lean on each other for support. I was completely unaware of the importance of self-care at this point in my life. I wasn't doing much of anything to take care of the health of my brain, as I am so fiercely committed to now.

When Mike returned, he received orders to Ft. Knox, and we moved back to Louisville—a dream come true. I retook the practical exam for my cosmetology license in Kentucky, found a salon job, and began planning my Aveda salon. Fear and doubt crept in, but a conversation with my best friend Robin renewed my resolve.

As we sat at the mall, she said, "If this is what you really want, I think you should do it." That moment solidified my decision to move forward. Little did I know, setting my intention would open doors I hadn't imagined, guiding me toward my dream salon.

Chapter 4

Fake It Til You Make It

When it came to opening my own salon, I had no idea where to start. With no nearby coffee shop to retreat to, I sat down at my kitchen table one day while Julia was at daycare. I was armed with a notebook and determined to put my business degrees to work. The problem was that, despite my education, neither of my degrees had taught me how to start a business from scratch. So, I turned to the internet for answers. I typed in searches like, *What are the steps to starting a business?* and *What do you need to start a business?* After a few searches and a lot of note-taking, I identified the main steps: create a business plan, find funding, secure a location, and get in contact with Aveda.

I found a few examples of business plans online and used them as templates for mine. I tried to include as much detail as possible about my vision, but starting a business from scratch meant a lot of unknowns. Much of what I wrote felt like a fairytale—an ideal scenario I hoped would come true. Aveda provided some preliminary revenue projections, but I hadn't yet hired staff or finalized a menu of services. How was I supposed to include financial projections when so much was still theoretical?

Once my business plan was complete, the next step was funding. As I often did when it came to money or business questions, I turned to my dad. He had banked with the same institution for more than 30 years and was still in touch with some of the loan officers, so he arranged for an introduction. On the day of the meeting, I dressed in my best business suit, ready with several spiral-bound copies of my business plan I had printed at Kinko's. *Dress for success*, I reminded myself.

My dad introduced me with confidence that I didn't yet feel: "This is my daughter, Laura. She wants to open a salon, and she needs some money." His straightforwardness made me smile as I shook hands with the bankers, nervous but determined.

I handed over copies of my business plan, feeling vulnerable as I watched them flip through my dreams in black and white. *What if they laugh at me? What if they think, 'Who does she think she is, asking for this much money?'* Thankfully, my fears didn't come true. They were impressed with my dual qualifications—an MBA and a cosmetology license—and appreciated the effort I had put into my plan. To my relief, I qualified for a Patriot Loan, a program for military personnel or their spouses who are starting a business. With my dad co-signing, I secured $65,000 in financing to start my salon.

For the location, I targeted an area of town with rapid residential growth but limited commercial development. There were no upscale salon-spa options in the area and no Aveda presence. It seemed like the perfect spot. As luck would have it, I found a space that had previously been a salon. It had closed nearly a year earlier, and still had useful equipment like shampoo bowls and a washer and dryer, which saved me some initial costs. After touring the space, the landlord and I scheduled a meeting to discuss the lease.

Walking into that meeting, I felt completely unprepared. *What do I know about signing a commercial lease?* I thought. *What am I even going to ask about?* The phrase *"fake it till you make it"* repeated in my head as I sat in the conference room waiting for the landlord, a seasoned businessman nearing retirement. He was polite and professional, and despite my nerves, I presented myself as confident. I even managed to negotiate a $15,000 build-out allowance, which I would repay at 7% interest over the course of the lease. The terms were good, especially considering the economy was tanking in 2008. Signing that lease felt monumental—equal parts terrifying and exhilarating.

Working with Aveda was another challenge. The approval process took four months and required submitting my business plan, proof of access to $250,000 in funding, and waiting for their internal board to review my application. Every day was a learning experience as I navigated meetings with bankers, landlords, and Aveda's development team. I felt vulnerable but determined. Failure was not an option, even though I knew the odds weren't in my favor—half of all small businesses fail in their first year.

Finally, on Saturday, November 22, 2008, Pure Salon Spa opened its doors. I had a full book of clients that day, five stylists, and a staff member on the front desk. Mike brought our daughter to visit, commenting that stress was written all over my face. He wasn't wrong. I didn't yet understand that to be a successful small business owner, I would have to learn to endure a level of stress that would crush most people. Nor had I learned that even *good stress*, that I actually *chose* to introduce into my life, if not dealt with properly could eventually cause me to develop a mental illness. I had convinced myself that the stress *I had chosen*, such as moving across the country, marrying a guy in the military, having children, or starting a business somehow didn't count. I felt like I shouldn't let it affect me as much as a stress that had been imposed on me unwillingly.

I realize now that a "failure is not an option" mentality is an incredible amount of pressure to place on yourself—equal parts good and bad. Good in ways that keep you inspired and driven to succeed. Bad in that unless you are able to balance it in a healthy way, eventually it can cause serious problems with your mental health. Back then, I should have created a self-care plan at the very same time I was creating my business plan. That stress would persist for years as I learned the realities of running a small business.

Owning a business is hard. People think it's glamorous, but in the beginning, the owner is the first to arrive, the last to leave, and the last to get paid. Every decision and every risk rests on your shoulders. I agonized over firing employees who weren't a good fit and took it personally when people quit. Leading a salon team is deeply personal work, requiring incredible heart, and often heartbreak. No one tells you about the sleepless nights, the family sacrifices, and the toll it takes on your marriage. It's soul-crushing at times, but with love, support, and sometimes therapy, you can push through.

Despite the challenges, Pure Salon Spa grew rapidly, even in the middle of a recession. By our third year, we were honored as one of the *Salon Today* Top 200 Salons in North America, a distinction we've received almost every year since 2011. Much of our success is thanks to Jennifer, the manager I hired early on, who had more industry experience than me. She's been instrumental in creating the systems and structure that make us successful to this day.

In the midst of growing the business, Mike and I welcomed our second daughter, Shelby, in 2010. Mike's final military assignment was approaching, and we decided I would remain in Louisville with the kids while he finished his last two years on active duty. We knew it wasn't ideal, but at least I would be at home surrounded by a tribe of support that could help me with the girls, while I again assumed the role of single parenting and grew my salon.

However, the Army had other plans—Mike unexpectedly received orders to deploy to Afghanistan for six months *before* his next assignment. I was furious. This wasn't part of our plan, and the thought of another deployment, especially in Afghanistan, was overwhelming. *Why does he have to go?* I wondered. He wasn't even attached to a unit that was deploying. To me, this felt like an attack on our family and on him that I couldn't quite come to terms with. I was furious at the army and furious at Mike, even though I knew I shouldn't be. As time went on, I let the anger consume me. I was hanging on by a thread mentally and refused to admit it.

Our oldest daughter, now seven, understood what was happening and was terrified of Mike's deployment. She had nightmares about her dad being killed and started struggling at school. I enrolled her in therapy, but juggling her needs, the salon, and raising two children alone was exhausting me. I coped poorly—overcommitting to business opportunities, going out too often to blow off steam, and constantly feeling guilty for not being there for my kids the way I wanted. I now see the irony of how quick I was to get Julia into therapy because I wanted to help her, while I ignored my own need for support. Why was it so natural to believe she deserved the best care but I had to handle everything alone?

During this period of time, I experienced a strange sensation while I was at one of Julia's swim meets—my brain felt like it was vibrating, and I became lightheaded. I pushed through, as always, telling myself to just keep going. But I realize now I was burning out, running on anger, guilt, and frustration. By the time Mike returned, I was an emotional wreck, disconnected from him and overwhelmed by the toll the deployment had taken on our marriage. For the first time, we weren't on the same page.

Chapter 5

Maybe You Should Pray More

Ultimately, Mike and I decided the best move for our family was for me and our girls to join him in San Antonio, Texas, at his final duty station. My salon manager, Jennifer, was capable of running Pure in my absence. The plan was for me to work remotely from Texas and commute back to Kentucky every couple months to check in on my team. The Army packed us up, we sold our house, and we embarked on what felt like an endless drive from Kentucky to Texas with two kids and a cat in tow.

While I was excited for a fresh start, fear weighed on me. This time, the fear wasn't about being alone in a new place while Mike deployed to a dangerous location. Instead, it was about leaving my business in someone else's hands. Although I trusted my manager, our move coincided with losing our top-performing stylist—a challenge I hadn't anticipated.

A few months before we moved to Texas, this stylist and I returned from what I thought was a dynamic presentation at a local cosmetology school.

As we settled back into work, she approached me. "Can I meet with you sometime today?" she asked.

"Sure thing," I replied, assuming she wanted my support with a new idea for driving revenue or another initiative in the salon. She was, and still is, one of the most passionate and driven stylists I have ever worked with. Under myself and Jennifer's coaching, she achieved more in a short amount of time than anyone else on my team, past or present. Her work ethic and enthusiasm were unmatched, and she had a remarkable ability to connect with people.

But when we sat down, her words blindsided me.

"I just wanted to let you know that I'm no longer going to be supporting your vision for Pure. It's time for me to work on my vision now, which is to open my own salon."

I was dumbfounded. I had naively assumed she would stick around for a few more years, given the fact she was thriving in the environment we had created.

Trying to collect myself, I asked, "How long have you been feeling this way?"

"For a while now," she replied, "so I thought I should go ahead and tell you, so you wouldn't be surprised when I left."

"When do you plan on leaving?" I questioned.

"I'd like to stay until the end of the year," she said.

Feeling desperate, I agreed to let her stay another four months. I thought this would delay the immediate loss of revenue and give me time to create a replacement plan. However, as weeks passed, the decision proved to be a mistake. I overheard her whispering to clients about her plans and I could feel the team's energy shifting. The tension in the salon was palpable.

Two weeks before our move to Texas, my manager approached me, her tone serious. "I can't do this with her until the end of the year," she said. "It's already weird and stressful, and I don't want to handle this alone while you're gone."

She was right, as she often is. As much as I wanted to avoid dealing with the situation before leaving, I had to support Jennifer.

We decided to move up the stylist's last day and communicate it to her as soon as possible. Since our space didn't have a private office, I dragged three chairs outside to the narrow strip of concrete behind the building, next to the AC unit. Then, I asked both women to step outside with me. Hardly ideal, but it was all we had.

"I'm getting ready to move to San Antonio," I began, "and Jennifer has concerns about navigating your exit without me here to support her. We've decided that your last day will be two weeks from today."

She was shocked, clearly not expecting to leave three months earlier than planned. Shaking her head, she muttered, "This is really shitty."

At the time, it probably was. I went back on our agreement. Looking back, I realize how naïve it was for me to let her "quit and stay" for four months while planning her own salon in my space. Years later, with more experience, I handled a similar situation very differently. Still, I knew I had made the right decision to back my manager and address the issue before moving.

Over the following months, I faced the fallout: many clients followed the stylist to her new salon, she opened a competing Aveda salon just 12 miles away, and I lost several team members to her. It was, indeed, a shitty situation.

We arrived in San Antonio and moved into a two-bedroom townhouse. Adjusting to a new city, Julia's new school, Shelby's new daycare, Mike's new job, and my new way of owning a business from afar was overwhelming. The gravity of our isolation hit me when I filled out Julia's school paperwork and realized I had no local emergency contact to list. It was just us.

Ever since the girls started school and daycare, we had always lived near friends, family, or a military community we could rely on. Now, we had no one. The thought of being unable to come to my children's rescue if something happened was terrifying. In the end,

Mike asked a colleague at work to serve as our emergency contact—a stranger, stepping in for my precious girls.

The guilt and anger came flooding in. *If I had held it together better while Mike was in Afghanistan, we wouldn't be in this situation. If I were a better mom, we wouldn't have had to move. If the Army hadn't sent Mike on that random deployment, we'd still be near friends and family.*

Though we eventually found our footing in San Antonio, there were a few big bumps in the road for me. After we were there awhile, I visited a nearby Air Force clinic for allergy issues. During the appointment, the doctor reviewed my chart and noticed I was on Lexapro.

"How long have you been taking this?" he asked.

When I explained why, his response floored me. "Do you and your husband go to church?" he asked.

Confused, I replied, "Sometimes."

"You may want to consider going to church more often and really praying about why you're anxious," he said. "Then you might not need Lexapro anymore."

I was stunned.

Wasn't I there to see him about my allergies? Did I ask for his opinion on my mental health?

I politely said, "You might be right." eager to end the appointment.

On the drive home, his words replayed in my mind. Had he really implied that my anxiety was a lack of faith? Was he suggesting I could pray away my mental health struggles? His comments made me feel ashamed for needing medication, even though I knew I shouldn't be. This was my first real experience with a medical professional perpetuating the stigma surrounding mental health and it left a bad taste in my mouth. Even with limited knowledge of mental health at the time, I knew his line of thinking was wrong. Now I know it wasn't just inappropriate—it was harmful.

It is alarming to think about the lack of knowledge that a lot of medical professionals still have surrounding mental health. Or those who don't think struggles of this type are valid medical conditions. The stigma that is associated with mental health is particularly dangerous because feeling like their struggles aren't real or justified keeps people from asking for the help they need. Untreated mental illness can be as life-threatening as a stroke, heart attack, or diabetes and should be taken seriously.

My mental health was deteriorating quickly during this time, but I didn't know it. Even though I was showing up for myself and my family and, in many cases, achieving a lot of success, I wasn't prioritizing my mental health. If that doctor had recognized that I was probably on Lexapro because I was struggling mentally and met me with some empathy about it, that would have changed my perspective.

Rather than implying that I could pray my way out of anxiety, it could have been an excellent opportunity for this doctor to find out more about me. Or even to introduce me to the concept of self-care or educate me on how the relentless pace I was keeping could affect me down the road. I would have been receptive and maybe even changed my lifestyle in ways that could have helped me avoid a mental health crisis.

Over time, living in San Antonio turned out to be a blessing. Mike and I grew closer with the help of marriage counseling, and our little family became tighter than ever. We immersed ourselves in Texas culture, met wonderful friends, and made new memories. I flew back to Louisville every eight weeks to check on Pure, juggling business, motherhood, and marriage as best as I could. It wasn't perfect, but it was progress.

Chapter 6

Beach Weekend

I woke up one of my last mornings in Texas with my head pounding and my mouth dry. I had to swallow a couple times to keep my tongue from sticking to the roof of my mouth. *Where is my chapstick?* I wondered as I struggled to turn on the bedside lamp. I knew I should have stopped at a couple of drinks the night before, but the conversation was flowing and this was one of the last weekends I would see this group of girls—my Texas friends.

We were at the beach in Port Aransas, Texas, for a girl's weekend. Sadly, our family's time living in San Antonio was coming to an end. My friends and I had fellowshipped, book clubbed, wine toured, backyard picnicked, and laughed a million laughs together. Still, I felt a heaviness from knowing in the next couple weeks we would be moving back to Louisville and, once again, leaving these friends behind.

The car ride home looked no different than any other times we had ridden somewhere together. My friends happily chatting away, reminiscing about the weekend, and talking about how sunny and beautiful the sky was, but the ride felt different to me. I couldn't quite put my finger on it because it was a feeling I had never felt before. Even though I brushed it off and tried to enjoy the rest of the ride, I was mostly stuck in my head wondering why I felt weird. Something just felt *off*.

The next couple of weeks went by in a blur. So many things to do, coordinate, and details to take care of. My husband was preparing for retirement from his 20-year army career and we were moving our family back to my hometown. I knew I was supposed to be excited. The army had already packed and moved our things a few days before we drove to Louisville, so we stayed in a hotel. I was trying to balance working, last minute phone calls to tie up loose ends, and shuttling my kids to and from school. It felt especially stressful and messy, but I shrugged it off. I thought it was just part of moving across the country and the bittersweetness of leaving another group of friends I had met through the military.

All the exciting things I had been dreaming about were happening. We were finally, after 13 years of moving around for Mike's career, going back to where everything was familiar. From reconnecting with friends and family, to purchasing the perfect home in an area of town where I had always wanted to live, and getting my girls into our chosen schools, this was supposed to be amazing. So why didn't it feel that way?

Our household goods arrived and we went to work unpacking the boxes. As we were putting dishes in the cabinets on one of the first nights in our new home, my husband asked, "What's wrong with you?"

"What do you mean?" I asked and stopped what I was doing, kind of annoyed with him.

"Why aren't you happier?" he went on, "We are finally done with all the moving around. I'm retiring, you are home with your friends and family and able to work in your salon every day if you want. So, why aren't you feeling happier?"

There it was.

I was wondering the same thing—why wasn't I happy? Mike

saw it, too. It was almost a relief when he said it out loud because I had been thinking it in my head. Since I first felt *it* the day I came home from the beach trip with the girls, I'd been fighting with myself. *Something felt off.* Even though I knew I should be feeling happy and excited, no matter how much I tried, I just didn't. I felt numb.

I tried to explain to him how I felt but it was so hard to put into words. None of the anxiety and mental discomfort made any sense to me, so how was I supposed to explain it to someone else? Luckily, I married the right guy who cares about my happiness, so he noticed. I felt a little better just trying to express to him how I was struggling, even though I didn't understand it yet.

We chalked my feelings up to the move, stress from starting a new chapter in our lives, and being overwhelmed. I didn't know it then, but it was the beginning of a new chapter alright—one that would last almost 10 years. This chapter would take me into a darkness like nowhere I've ever been. This is a darkness nobody talks about openly because there is still so much stigma around depression and mental health issues. Something "feels off" was a big understatement. In the coming months and years, I would begin to understand exactly why.

Mike's retirement wasn't official until the Fall of 2015, but we wanted the girls to start fresh at the beginning of a new school year in Kentucky. This meant I was living in our new house solo with the girls for a few months before he moved home permanently. After all of the unpacking was finished, Mike headed back to San Antonio for work. This wasn't my first rodeo with a scenario like this. Although difficult, I always made it through bouts of solo parenting, adjusting to moves, and being away from Mike just fine before.

This time was different because of the toll the transition was taking on my mental health. I grew increasingly anxious about things I had never worried about before. I would agonize over simple decisions like what to have for dinner and would yearn for bedtime, so I could break down and cry in the privacy of our bedroom. I didn't want the girls to see how sad and anxious I was. Tears became my only release.

Constant negative self-talk began to haunt my every waking moment. I went through the motions of life, but if anyone snuck a peek inside my thoughts, they would have been amazed at the war in my head. I woke up every day feeling exhausted and got really good at faking it and smiling through my pain.

One weekend, while Mike was still in Texas, I remember taking the girls to my mom's for the afternoon. We had lunch and it was a beautiful day. My mom had something delicious prepared for us, as she always does, and I played along with the small talk. I was feeling nervous and paranoid she might uncover that something was *really* wrong with me.

At one point, the girls went outside to play. My mom started cleaning up the kitchen and I couldn't hold it in any longer.

"Mom," my voice trembled as the tears started to fall, "I'm not okay." That was as honest as I could be at the time and I know it made absolutely no sense to her.

In her kind, nurturing way, she stopped what she was doing, sat down with me at the table and asked, "What's wrong?"

"I don't even know how to explain it, but I feel like I'm losing my mind," I said. She looked at me with concern as I continued, "I can't get control of my thoughts. I feel anxious and worried all the time." She stared at me waiting for me to continue but all I could do was cry.

"Well honey," she offered, "you are handling a lot right now and I know that can be overwhelming, but you'll get through this like you always have." She spoke soothingly and assured me I had her support with whatever I needed.

Even though I appreciated what she had to say and knew it was true, it wasn't enough. I felt just a little bit of relief, like a pot of simmering water that had finally boiled over. The water level had lowered a little, but only temporarily. Until the heat rose and the water boiled over again. For the next several weeks, I lived on the edge of boiling over. It was scary, frustrating, embarrassing, and uncomfortable. I would boil over and cry multiple times a day, feeling temporary relief. Then the process would repeat.

This went on for several months until my primary care doctor finally suggested I see a psychiatrist.

"I feel like what you're experiencing is beyond my realm of expertise and I want you to see a specialist." she told me during a visit.

At that point I didn't know the difference between a psychiatrist, a psychologist, or a therapist but she explained to me that a psychiatrist works specifically with mental illnesses that affect the brain.

How presumptuous of her to think I'm mentally ill! I thought to myself. *Does she think I'm crazy? I'm NOT crazy! How can someone like me be mentally ill?*

During the period of time I was working with my primary physician, my depression and anxiety symptoms persisted and got much worse. I started to learn that mental health treatment can be like a guessing game. Figuring out which medications work on what symptoms and the process of weaning off medications, while simultaneously introducing new ones to your system, is long and excruciating. Especially when you're struggling.

Each time I started a new medication I was so hopeful that THIS ONE would make me feel better. I was in a constant state of waiting and suffering. If a medication happened to work, it was only temporary. Inevitably, I would drag myself back into the doctor's office to explain, once again, that I was experiencing failure. I knew it was actually the medication failing, but the evil inside my head convinced me that *I* was failing. Every time a medication stopped working, I would have panic attacks until I just couldn't take it anymore. When I finally told someone, I was embarrassed about being unable to control my emotions. I cried like a baby, trying to explain why I was upset, while my loved ones reacted in helpless disbelief, not knowing how to help me.

At first, I would only share my struggles with my husband or my mom because I was too ashamed. After all, I thought I had a reputation to uphold—badass business woman, salon owner, mother, and wife. If you were on the outside looking in on my life, you would think I had it made, baby! I kept asking myself what the hell I had to be anxious or depressed about. I worried that people would think I was crazy or ungrateful or just being dramatic.

The thought of seeing a specialist gave me some hope. Since my primary care doctor wasn't able to figure this out, I figured maybe a psychiatrist would have the magic answer. I started on the hunt for a psychiatrist and chose one based on some recommendations. At the first appointment I found him to be professional and thorough but not very personable. As I sat in his office across from him, I answered basic questions and did my best to explain the events that led me there. He took notes, nodded, and seemed to process everything I was telling him. It felt so vulnerable to be relaying the deepest, darkest secrets of my soul to a stranger. He couldn't know who I really was as a person, what I had achieved in my life, or even how desperate I was for him to help me.

"Well Laura," he began, "It sounds like you're experiencing Major Depressive Disorder."

There it is! I thought. *I finally have a name and a cause for what I'm feeling!*

The psychiatrist immediately began discussing the medication he was going to prescribe, which was Trintellex. Not once did he ask me about how much alcohol I drank, my eating habits, or if and how much I exercised. The entire experience was very clinical and felt absent of any kind of human touch or empathy. Despite this, I decided to proceed. After all, he was the expert and that's what my primary doctor said I needed.

While I understand the need for a clinical approach to medicine, it would have been a game-changer, as I sobbed in my initial evaluation with the psychiatrist, if he had simply said: *"This is not your fault. What you are feeling is the result of an imbalance in your brain chemistry. In order to provide you relief from these symptoms, we need to find the right combination of medications and treatments that will bring balance to your brain. This may take some time but we will get there. In addition to traditional medication and treatment, let's dive into some other areas of your life that could also be affecting your mental health."*

Maybe he assumed I understood more than I actually did about mental illness or what had landed me in his office. This assumption was dangerous because I didn't have a clue what was happening to me. Much less, that what I was experiencing all boiled down to brain chemistry. I didn't yet understand how the internalized stigma that existed around mental health was impacting my experience. Had that doctor attempted to educate and assure me, I would have been grateful. It may have saved me from the shame and guilt I felt.

When I finally mustered the courage to find a mental health provider, that first appointment was crucial. It set the stage for the entire recovery process. I had already experienced judgement and criticism from a different medical professional about being on a medication for anxiety. It would have helped me so much if a doctor had explained the basic neuroscience—the *why*—behind what was happening to me. Maybe even given me a rough idea of what the process of healing might look like. It may have silenced the self-doubt and unrelenting voice of criticism I placed on myself. On some level, I still thought I could somehow *will* my way out of feeling depressed.

For the next two years, I endured a roller-coaster of starting new medications filled with hope and waiting weeks to see if they worked. Some worked, some didn't—and when they stopped, the cycle repeated. Each time a medication failed, I felt more like I was the failure. At one point, my doctor even prescribed Lithium. *Lithium?* I knew then I had officially entered the depths of mental illness. Then, at my last visit, he suggested ECT—Electroconvulsive Therapy.

"If I were in your shoes, I'd do ECT," he said. "You run a business—you don't have time to waste. This would be the fastest way to recovery."

While all of these things were true, he shared very little information with me about the procedure beyond his opinion. I was left wondering what ECT entailed, how many others he had referred to the treatment, or whether this doctor had any consideration for what I was actually comfortable with as the patient. His recommendation felt like more of a demand than a suggestion. I got the sense he was losing patience with me. For someone who was supposed to be an expert on "feelings" he had completely missed the mark.

I refused ECT immediately—it sounded terrifying. And his flippant attitude about it pissed me off. At the end of the visit, I asked for other options. He mentioned TMS (Transcranial Magnetic Stimulation) and Ketamine Infusions. As soon as I got home, I started researching my treatment options and new psychiatrists.

Because I'd had enough of this guy.

Chapter 7

California Rocket Fuel

I have always dreamed of being a business coach for other salon owners, and in August 2018, I had the opportunity to attend a Strategies coaching certification in New Haven, Connecticut. I had worked with Strategies and adopted their team-based pay model in my salon in 2015, which compelled me to pursue coaching with them.

When the opportunity presented itself, I was on new medication and feeling good about my mental health, so I decided to go for it. The certification required a $5,000 investment, several days of training, and, at the end, a test to assess everything we had learned. The highest scorer on the test would earn the opportunity to attend a future workshop at Strategies' education center and present their experience transitioning to team-based pay.

I was excited about the possibility of presenting. And because I am a star student—and let's not forget, an overachiever—I aced the test, earning the highest score in my class.

Yes! Woohoo! I thought when my score was revealed. *This will be my chance to start teaching other salon owners what I've learned! It's a foot in the door to begin coaching with an incredible company in the beauty industry.*

At the same time, a sinking feeling crept in. A voice in my head reminded me that I was mentally ill, and my depression could sabotage my plans if this medication stopped working—just like so many others had before. When I got home and returned to the salon, my team had written notes of congratulations and signed the back of a "Boss" sign meant for my desk—a daily reminder of what I had accomplished. They all knew how important coaching was to me, and it felt incredible to have their support, knowing they were proud of me.

I hoped like hell I could continue making them proud, following through with this opportunity, and that my depression wouldn't ruin it for me. I pushed forward, working on my presentation for the upcoming workshop where I would be a speaker. I practiced with the education leader at Strategies—an intimidating guy with a big personality who, if I'm being honest, I was a little afraid of.

As the weeks led up to my travel date, I started to spiral. The cycle was beginning again. I could feel the symptoms of depression creeping in, but I was in denial.

Nope. It's not happening again. I will not let this get in the way of what I've been working toward and dreaming of.

How naïve I was about mental health back then—thinking I could control the sickness in my brain simply by willing it away. It's almost funny now, how ridiculous that notion was. And yet, so many people still don't understand mental health enough to realize that when your brain is sick, no amount of telling yourself to *feel better* or *act right* is going to fix it. If it worked that way, we could end so much suffering. We could eliminate suicide, ensure no one ever had to miss out on opportunities to chase their dreams, lose their jobs, or be hospitalized just because their brain chemistry was off.

As the weeks leading up to my presentation passed, I kept sinking lower and lower. Two days before I was supposed to travel, my anxiety reached an all-time high. Even though I wasn't ready to admit it, there was no way I could pull this off in my current mental state. The night before my flight to Strategies for my presentation, I was scheduled to chaperone my youngest daughter's Girl Scout overnight trip. I desperately wanted to cancel, but there was no way I would disappoint her like that. So, I put on my brave face, and we went.

It was excruciating trying to appear okay in front of the other moms, the kids, and—most importantly—my own daughter. I knew how embarrassed she would be if I broke down in tears or bailed on the experience entirely. I somehow managed to get through it, but I didn't sleep at all that night. Extreme panic had set in, and I spent the night trapped in a mental battle between two opposing voices in my head.

One voice told me to suck it up, put on my big girl panties, get on that plane, and deliver the presentation like I had committed to. The other voice insisted there was absolutely no way I could do this on my own without completely embarrassing myself—and if I did, my secret mental health struggles would be out in a community I was desperately trying to prove myself to.

When we arrived home, I was exhausted, and my anxiety was mounting. I had about four hours before my flight to the presentation, and the reality was setting in—I wasn't going. My opportunity to speak and become a coach wasn't going to happen. I headed upstairs to pack, but instead, I started crying. My thoughts were racing. Even though I knew what I had to do, I had no idea how to go about it. The familiar shame spiral had begun.

How in the world do I cancel this trip with Strategies and let them know I can't come—without telling them I'm mentally ill? If I'm honest, what will they think of me? They'll think I'm a flake, irresponsible—probably relieved they dodged a bullet by not continuing this process with me. That's what. Because I'm unreliable and crazy and have no business representing them or coaching other salon owners. Who was I kidding? I'm ridiculous. A fraud. How embarrassing this must be for my family—

this weakness I can't control. I'm a joke. And now, they'll really know it when I mess this up. This was my chance, and I've blown it.

It took everything I had to walk back downstairs to my husband. Before I knew it, I was sobbing.

"I can't do it," I said as he turned around to see what was happening.

"I'm a freaking mess. I can't stop crying, and there is absolutely no way I can travel and get through this presentation. I have to cancel, but I'm afraid to call and tell them. Will you help me?"

"Are you sure?" he asked, but he already knew the answer. He could see me falling apart.

"Positive," I said.

"Well, I think you're going to have to call them and let them know you aren't coming." He said seriously.

Those were the words I didn't want to hear, even though I knew that was what needed to happen. We sat down together, and I wrote out what to say.

This was a medical emergency—I was literally falling apart, mentally and emotionally. But because of the stigma surrounding mental health, it didn't *feel* like I could call it an emergency. I mean, sure, if I were having chest pains or slurred speech, that would be an emergency everyone would understand. But would they accept this?

Would they judge me? Be angry that I was canceling at the last minute?

As I dialed the number of the guy who had been helping me prepare my presentation, my heart was racing. My breathing grew faster, and before I knew it, I was in a full-blown panic attack just as he answered.

"Hello," he said.

"Hi. This is Laura." My voice was frantic, my thoughts scattered. I was crying, and I knew he could hear the panic in my voice.

"There has been an emergency, and I'm not going to be able to make it there to present." I forced myself to say.

Silence. He was processing what I had just said.

"...Okay?" he responded, uncertain.

"I'm really sorry, and I'll get back in touch when I can."

He asked, "Is everything okay?" but I barely registered it.

"Not really," I admitted, "but I can't talk now. I just wanted to let you know I wasn't coming."

I'm sure he was confused and concerned for my well-being, but I was too embarrassed to explain what was really going on. I'm sure I sounded like a frazzled mess, offering him almost no information, only shame and panic.

What I wished I could have said was:

Hi, this is Laura, and I'm so very sorry to have to cancel my trip this weekend. I'm currently in a full-blown panic attack as I tell you this, and I'm in the middle of a crisis with my mental health. I am terribly embarrassed and hate myself for letting you down, but this is completely out of my control, and I need to make a choice that is best for me right now. I realize how this looks, and I feel awful that I am letting you and the rest of the participants down. Please forgive me. I hope you'll give me another chance in the future when I've figured out a solution to my anxiety and depression.

Instead, I got off the phone as quickly as I could, avoiding further questions and humiliation. I left him hanging, wondering what the hell had just happened. As soon as I hung up, I broke down. I cried so hard I couldn't catch my breath, hyperventilating until my body finally gave out from exhaustion. And then, once I calmed down, the shame spiral started.

The monster inside my head was relentless.

You're a failure.

Sure, I had escaped the burden of travel and public speaking, but now I had left them wondering *what happened* to me. I had only bought myself a couple of days before I would have to come up with an explanation—one that made sense, one that they would *accept*.

What could I tell them that wouldn't make me sound crazy?

I tried to sleep, but it was useless. The voice in my head wouldn't let me rest. It kept reminding me that my reputation was ruined. That I had just kissed this coaching opportunity goodbye.

And once again, the medication was failing. That meant another round of doctor's appointments, admitting yet another failure.

I felt completely defeated. Embarrassed.

After a couple of years and in a much healthier mental space, I reached back out to Strategies to explain what had happened in full transparency. I was met with so much care and compassion in their response and it helped me realize that mental health struggles are more common than I thought.

Most people have struggled or know someone who has. Many others have suffered in silence because of the stigma. It is my hope that in the future, we are all met with care and compassion when we are brave enough to share our struggles in both personal and professional conversations. My experience with Strategies was not a waste of time or a complete failure like I thought at the time. Even though it didn't turn out like I expected, it was a learning experience in several ways. It taught me the concept of grace; giving it to myself and to others when things don't go as planned or take an unexpected turn that at first feels disappointing. It made me realize that having to say "no" to something doesn't always mean you don't want it bad enough. Sometimes, it's just the best you can do in that moment and it doesn't have to define your future.

Soon after, I found a new psychiatrist's office that specialized in Transcranial Magnetic Stimulation (TMS) and scheduled a consultation. I had to wait a couple of weeks for my appointment, but I went in with a renewed sense of hope—maybe TMS would be the answer.

The first appointment felt familiar, just like every other time I had met with a new doctor.

"Tell me why you're here, Laura," he said.

"I'm severely depressed and have tried so many medications that haven't worked. I'm still scared to try ECT, and I'm hoping maybe TMS is the answer," I responded, more questioning than explaining.

We discussed all the medications I had tried unsuccessfully. He went over my medical history and explained how TMS worked, including the success rates other patients had experienced. After our conversation, I decided to move forward, which meant I had to return to have my brain mapped. This process would determine the exact placement on my head for the magnet therapy I was about to start.

TMS seemed like a less terrifying option than ECT, even though it required a 30-minute session, five days a week for six weeks, just to see if it would make a difference. Each session involved sitting in a chair—similar to one at the dentist's office—while a piece of equipment was positioned close to the left side of my head. Once the treatment started, I felt a tapping sensation from the device, which used magnet therapy to stimulate the part of my brain that controlled mood.

According to the doctor, many patients had experienced significant success with TMS, finding relief from depression and anxiety. I prayed during every single 30-minute session that this would be the answer for me.

Those six weeks felt endless. Since I couldn't drive after the appointments, I had to rely on my family to take me each time. With every prayer, I wasn't just praying for myself—I was praying for them, too. Praying that they wouldn't have to take care of me anymore. It felt like too much of a burden, even though they never complained. They always showed up when I needed them. But as the weeks went on, I felt no relief. No improvement. Nothing.

It was heartbreaking.

Each week, I met with the doctor to discuss my progress, and each time, I had to admit to him that it wasn't working. That I felt no different than when I started. And with every one of those conversations, the shame weighed heavier on me. It wasn't the treatment that was failing—I was.

By my last session, I sat in front of the doctor, completely defeated, almost begging him for a next step.

"It's been six weeks, and I feel no different," I said. "What else can I try other than ECT?"

"Well," he began, "you may want to give Ketamine infusions a try. There's been some success with that in depressed patients, and it would be an alternative to ECT."

I left his office and went home—back to square one. Back to searching for a solution to my major depressive disorder. I felt so defeated. I had no idea where I would find the strength to keep going in this fight.

But by some miracle, I did.

Along the way, a friend mentioned that we had a mutual acquaintance, John, who had also struggled with depression. She told me he really liked his medical provider and encouraged me to give him a call. I wasn't sure what direction to take after finishing my TMS treatments, and I knew I didn't want to go back to my first psychiatrist, who insisted on ECT. So, I figured it wouldn't hurt to reach out and ask John who he was seeing. Maybe that could be a starting point.

John was a business acquaintance I knew through my banking relationships. At first, I was reluctant to call him. After all, I had a reputation to uphold as a businesswoman. Did I really want to open this can of worms with him? Not knowing where else to turn, I dialed his number.

"Hey, John," I started, my voice uncertain. "This is Laura

Watkins. You might remember me from when I opened my salon, and I'm also a friend of Samantha's."

"Hey, Laura," he said cheerfully, completely at ease.

I hesitated. What was I supposed to say next?

"I'm not sure if Samantha has shared this with you, but I'm really struggling right now with my mental health. She said you might have a provider you could recommend."

The next few seconds seemed to hang in eternity. I held my breath, dying of embarrassment, waiting for his response. This was the critical moment in a conversation like this—the moment where stigma and shame try to convince you that you've just made a terrible mistake. First, this was a call I never thought I'd have to make. To a person I never thought I'd have to call. About a subject I was still so deeply ashamed of. Second, John had only known me as the successful salon owner down the street. This could go one of two ways: he would meet my request with empathy and compassion or he would judge me—think I was crazy for calling, or worse, see me differently forever.

So much was at stake.

In the seconds before he spoke, I imagined myself blurting out, *Never mind, John, forget I called—just go back to thinking I'm a badass business owner.*

But what he said next put me on a path that would ultimately save my life.

"I know a lot about that, Laura, and I really hate to hear that you're suffering. I'm happy to help," he said.

His words hit me like a lifeline.

"I see a mental health nurse practitioner at a place called The Couch. It's kind of like an urgent care for mental health. She has really helped me find the right medications to manage my depression. Her name is Danielle, and I'd definitely recommend making an appointment with her."

We chatted a bit more, sharing our experiences with depression, and by the time I hung up, I felt something I hadn't felt in a long time: grateful. Grateful that I had called him. Grateful that he had answered with kindness.

John and I still keep in touch to this day. We have a silent understanding between us—a deep, unspoken acknowledgment of what it means to fight depression. How dark it can get. How hard we have to fight to keep it at bay.

A few days later, I had my first appointment with Danielle.

She listened intently as I described my symptoms, which had shifted from anxiety to mostly depression at that point. I walked her through the long list of medications I had tried and failed over the past three years and shared my experience with TMS, which, unfortunately, had shown no benefit for me.

Her notes from that first visit painted a stark picture:

Laura reports that she can get caught in a loop of worry. She states that she notices negative thoughts creeping in and becoming obsessive. She begins to isolate, avoiding phone calls from friends and family, who eventually notice and call it to her attention.

Laura reports impaired work performance and has not been to work in several weeks.

The patient describes the following depressive symptoms:

Sadness, tearfulness, emptiness, difficulty staying asleep, decreased interest and pleasure in daily activities, decreased appetite, weight loss, feelings of hopelessness, decreased energy, feelings of guilt and worthlessness, and suicidal thoughts.

Reading her notes was like seeing my pain laid out in black and white—clinical, factual, undeniable.

Medications patient has tried and failed:
Lexapro – Sept 2015 – May 2016
Effexor – July – November 2016
Trintellix – November 2016 – October 2017
Abilify – April – October 2017
Cymbalta – October 2017 – April 2018

Rexulti – November – April 2018
Nortriptyline – May 2018 – November 2018
Lithium – October – November 2018
Latuda – November 2018

I felt like I was in good hands with Danielle and trusted her plan for me. She recommended trying a combination of Trintellix and Abilify, along with Trazodone to help me sleep.

Sleep is crucial—for so many reasons, but especially for someone struggling with mental health. Sleep is the only time your brain gets a break from obsessive, negative thoughts and worry. Ironically, those same thoughts are often what keep you from falling asleep in the first place. Danielle also suggested I schedule an appointment with my primary care doctor to check my vitamin D levels—something none of my previous providers had ever mentioned.

Why the hell not?

She also recommended GeneSight testing, a simple test that identifies how a patient's genes can affect their response to medications commonly prescribed for depression. It provides information about which medications might require dosage adjustments, which are less likely to be effective, and which could have an increased risk of side effects based on genetic makeup.

Again—why the hell not?

These were basic but critical steps that had never been suggested to me before. Danielle seemed thorough, like she was starting with foundational elements that could make a huge difference in my recovery. I was relieved by that. And also pissed off. After three years of battling major depressive disorder, why had no one ever suggested these things? Shouldn't we have covered all of these bases by now?

Danielle also reiterated something I already knew but had conveniently ignored—alcohol was *not* recommended for someone struggling like I was. Alcohol fuels anxiety. It's a depressant. So, duh—maybe I shouldn't be drinking it?

This wasn't the first time I had heard this. One of my neighbors had recently stopped drinking and told me it had really helped with her crippling anxiety—among other things.

Maybe it was time I really listened.

By the time I met with Danielle again, my symptoms had improved. There was no way to know whether it was due to the new combination of medications she had prescribed or a delayed response to TMS—which I was told could also be the case.

I had also met with my primary physician, who ran a simple blood test and found that I was Vitamin D deficient—a condition that can contribute to mental illness. I immediately started taking a Vitamin D supplement along with my other medications.

Who knew?

At that point, *who cared?*

Because, for the first time in a long time, I felt somewhat normal. I was able to work again. But the relief came with an undercurrent of anxiety.

How long would this last?

My journey with mental health had started more than three years before, and by now, I had been through so many cycles—each one painfully familiar. The cycle always started with uneasiness and despair. Then, hope—hope that a new medication or treatment would work. Maybe it would work. Maybe temporarily. Then it wouldn't. I would admit another defeat, and the cycle would start all over again.

After enough of these cycles, even in the moments when I felt better, I couldn't enjoy it. Instead of relief, I developed a new worry—one that kept me from fully embracing the "better" moments.

I found myself waiting for the next crash. I avoided committing to anything new, afraid that I would eventually have to embarrass myself again—backing out, canceling, or failing because I would inevitably spiral back down into darkness. It wasn't fair—not to me, and not to the people around me who watched with fear, waiting for the inevitable. Because it always happened. I was desperate for a solution and fighting like hell to find one.

This was uncharted territory for me in every way. Not only was mental health new to me, but so was the feeling of being unable to achieve something I so desperately wanted for myself. I don't know which is worse: Going after something and not getting it? Or keeping myself from going after something because I know I won't be able to keep it? My resilience was being tested in a way it had never been before. And I was so damn tired of fighting.

By August 2019, my depressive symptoms had returned in full force. When I met with Danielle, I expressed my frustration. I wasn't feeling any better. I was struggling to go to work, make decisions, focus, or find energy. On top of that, I was waking up several times a night, trapped in relentless worry.

I brought up the idea of Ketamine infusions, and Danielle offered to have a medical assistant in her office do some research—gathering information about its benefits and how it had worked for other patients before making a recommendation.

Her visit notes that day included something that caught my eye: *Consider California Rocket Fuel (Effexor + Remeron)*.

At the time, I had no idea what that meant.

But later, I learned that California Rocket Fuel is a drug cocktail commonly prescribed for patients with treatment-resistant major depressive disorder—specifically for those who have tried multiple medications and failed to find relief.

Along with that, Danielle requested a follow-up test based on my original GeneSight results. This test would check for a variation in my MTHFR gene, which predicts a patient's ability to convert folic acid into its active form. Apparently, variations in the MTHFR gene and an inability to process folic acid can be linked to depression—something no previous provider had ever mentioned to me.

As it turns out, I *do* have an MTHFR mutation—or, as I now refer to it, my motherfucker gene.

Because of that, I now take a daily Methylfolate supplement as well.

By my next appointment with Danielle in October, I had been taking Vitamin D and Methylfolate regularly. I had also endured six Ketamine infusions—each one a failure, with no improvement whatsoever. The frustration I had felt at my last appointment had now morphed into disappointment and hopelessness.

Tearfully, I asked, "I am going to get better eventually, aren't I?"

At that point, I hadn't been to work in weeks. I had zero motivation, no ability to concentrate, no energy, and I was starting to give up. The mental pain and anguish were unbearable, and whatever hope I had left for recovery was fading.

I wanted to die.

My thoughts were consumed with one plan—the plan to end the pain myself.

What day will I pull into the garage and close the door behind me?

Who will find me?

I hope it's Mike and not one of the kids.

This is really going to be hard for them.

I hope they know I tried. I fought as long as I could.

This isn't because I don't love them. I love them so much... but this is just too painful to go on.

I am weaker than I thought.

And I can't take this anymore.

In my eyes, there was only one more thing left to try. And since I had already resolved to killing myself, ECT couldn't do any worse damage to me than that.

Chapter 8

The Lights Come Back On

The alarm sounded at 5 a.m. and immediately, I felt the familiar pit in my stomach. I had tossed and turned all night, dreading what was about to happen today, and now it was actually time to go. Thinking about it had made my anxiety so overwhelming that, in a twisted way, it almost balanced out my depression. Well...almost. Not really.

I was sick with worry over all the "what ifs."

What if this doesn't work, and there's nothing else left to try? What if I have to live in this misery for the rest of my life? What if something goes wrong, and I have a heart attack on the table? I mean, it is an electric current shooting through my body—what if my other major organs don't like that and decide to shut down? What if I wake up and my entire catalogue of memories is wiped clean, and I don't recognize my friends or family?

This relentless cycle of questioning had been looping in my head for days, and yet, despite my fear, I was desperate. I had tried what felt like a million other treatments, and nothing had given me the relief I needed to actually *live* among the living again. The alternative was incomprehensible. I couldn't fathom living another day the way I had been feeling, much less the rest of my life. I had decided that if this didn't work, I would kill myself to end the pain—despite always telling everyone who asked that I would never hurt myself.

It was still dark outside when we got in the car and started the drive to the hospital for my first of six ECT treatments. I was scared to death. Mike was driving, but I was trapped in my own head, consumed by worry. I don't think we spoke a single word to each other the whole way there; we were both lost in anticipation of what the day would bring. As we turned onto the long driveway leading up to the hospital, the reality of what I was about to do started to sink in. Still silent, Mike parked the car, and we walked toward the entrance together.

The doors were locked. Unlike a regular hospital, where you could just step up and trigger the automatic doors to slide open, this was a *mental* hospital—a place where people were treated for mental illness and substance abuse. That kind of freedom didn't exist here. It was so early, so dark, that if I hadn't known for certain I was supposed to arrive at this time for my treatment, I would have assumed the facility was closed. There was none of the usual activity of a "normal" hospital—no doors opening and closing, no people coming and going, no voices over an intercom. Just darkness and silence.

Through the glass doors, I could see a dimly lit waiting room, but no one was there to greet us. Just a crumpled old piece of paper flapping against a metal box, taped there instructing patients to dial 0 for the operator. The box creaked open as I reached for the cold phone, and I couldn't help but wonder how many other people had stood here in the darkness, doing the exact same thing.

"The Brook Hospital, how may I help you?" a voice answered.

"My name is Laura Watkins, and I have an appointment for ECT," I said weakly into the receiver.

"One moment, please. Someone will be there shortly to let you in."

A few minutes later, a hospital worker unlocked the door and led us inside to the waiting room. The large space was mostly empty, except for a few others who had arrived before me with their drivers.

Sitting there, my heart pounded so hard I had to remind myself to breathe. My palms were sweating. One by one, my fellow ECT patients and I emerged from the darkness, gathering in this sterile room, waiting for whatever came next.

I don't remember much about the others that day—except for one young girl who couldn't have been more than 20 years old. I remember thinking how heartbreaking it was that she needed such an aggressive treatment at such a young age. Her mother was with her, reeking of cigarettes, coughing with a deep, hacking rasp. I couldn't help but wonder what their story was. What had led them to this place?

We were all different—women, men, young, old. It struck me as ironic. Before this, I had never heard of anyone else undergoing ECT, and I hadn't told many people about it myself. Yet here we were, strangers bound together by a silent, shared understanding of what it felt like to be trapped in a mind that refused to function properly.

It was in that moment that I fully realized: mental illness doesn't discriminate. It isn't just for the "crazy" people—the ones you see on the streets, half-naked, screaming at a telephone pole. No. That's not necessarily what mental illness looks like. It can happen to *anyone*. At *any time*. No matter what kind of life they come from.

"Good morning," a nurse announced, and my heart jumped into my throat. "I'm here to take you down to ECT."

I stood up, and tears welled in my eyes. For a split second, I wanted to scream, *No! Stop! I've changed my mind. I can't do this. I'm too afraid*. But like most of the conversations I had been having in my head for years, I kept it to myself. Instead, I fell in line with the rest of the patients and followed the nurse to the elevator.

It felt eerily fitting that we rode the elevator *down* to the basement. We walked down a hallway, turned a corner, and came to a door labeled ECT. I half expected to walk into some kind of mad scientist's lab, complete with wild-haired doctors in white coats. Instead, we were greeted by two nurses in scrubs. They assigned us each a hospital bed and handed us clipboards with paperwork to complete.

One by one, we were called up for the routine check-in. The nurse took my blood pressure, verified my information and medications, and asked the standard question:

"Have you had any thoughts of hurting yourself or others?"

In all the years I've had ECT treatments, I've never heard a single person answer that question honestly. We *all* say no. And we *all* lie. In the darkest days of my depression, I used to wake up every morning hoping I would die in a car accident. But every time I was asked that question, I always said no.

The nurse found my vein without any trouble and injected a medication that slowed saliva production so I wouldn't choke on my own spit during the treatment. Then came another medication to combat the inevitable headache I would wake up with afterward.

Now what? I wondered.

I was prepped and ready, my heart still pounding in my chest, and I was still contemplating making a run for it. Thinking, *if I got up now, I could find my way back to the waiting room and beg Mike to take me home.* But before I acted on that impulse, a familiar voice interrupted my thoughts.

"Hi, Laura. It's good to see you again," said Dr. Burke. "How has your depression been?"

I glanced at him and noticed the faint red lines across his face, leading to the back of his head—the unmistakable marks from a CPAP machine. It was so early that his skin hadn't had time to smooth them out.

For a brief second, I wanted to say, *Dude, I think you already know. I'm here to get my brain zapped—how do you think my depression has been?* But I don't get snarky. I swallowed my sarcasm because I needed to believe that this man—this doctor—had the knowledge and skill to make me well again, even though several others in his profession had failed.

I wondered what it must feel like to hold that kind of power. To know you can pull someone back from the depths of despair. Someone who has spiraled down, down, down into a darkness so unbearable that they're inches away from shutting the garage door and starting the car.

"Looks like you'll be next," he said before moving on to check in with the next patient.

The next thing I knew, the metal brakes on my hospital bed clanged free, and I was being rolled into the treatment room. I focused on my breathing, tried to stay calm, but I was failing miserably.

A tall, white-haired man in scrubs, who reminded me of Captain Kangaroo, approached and explained that he'd be placing an oxygen mask near my head. Another nurse stuck electrodes to my chest, arms, and legs, connecting them to an ECG machine by thin lead wires. The machine would monitor my heart's electrical activity while the ECT was administered.

My fear resurfaced. *What if my heart stops? What if it explodes right here on the table?* But it was too late to back out now. I decided to let the experts take over and prayed like hell that this worked.

Then, out of the corner of my eye, I spotted something on the counter—a Styrofoam bite guard. My stomach turned. *I know what that's for.* They were going to shove it in my mouth before the electricity surged through my brain, forcing my body into convulsions. It would keep me from chipping a tooth or, worse, swallowing my tongue.

"Here comes some sleeping medicine," Captain Kangaroo announced as he pushed something magical into my IV.

A metallic taste bloomed in my mouth, and within seconds, I drifted into peaceful oblivion.

I came to slowly, my mind groggy but intact. Voices murmured around me. I was relieved to recognize where I was, who I was, and what just happened. My vision cleared, and everything seemed... normal. Except for the dull, aching sensation in my head—something I'd never felt before.

It was over. I survived.

But as the fog lifted, an all-too-familiar sensation crept in: the weight of my depression, still sitting heavy in my chest. *What if this is just another failed treatment?* A wave of desperation washed over me.

A nurse approached. "How are you feeling?" she asked as she removed my IV.

I heard her pick up the phone. "Hi, Mike? This is Francen in the ECT department. Laura is ready if you want to pull around and pick her up."

She turned back to me and helped me into a wheelchair.

But wait, Francen! I'm not ready! I'm not fixed yet, so how can I be ready?

I screamed the words inside my head, but no one heard. No one ever did. Instead, I stayed quiet as she rolled me down the hall, out into the early morning light.

Mike was waiting by the car. The nurse handed him a clipboard, barely acknowledging me as she went over post-treatment instructions.

"She might have a headache today, which can be treated with Tylenol as needed. Because she was under anesthesia, she can't drive or operate heavy machinery for 24 hours," she explains. "She should avoid making any important decisions or signing legal documents for the next several days. Normal activities can resume within a few hours if she feels up to it. She may experience nausea, muscle aches, confusion, and some short-term memory loss. That's normal and should subside within a few days. However, if she experiences severe pain, shortness of breath, chest pain, or a fast heartbeat, call us immediately."

I'm right here! I wanted to scream. *I'm not invisible!*

But I didn't.

Instead, I let them move me like a lifeless doll, from the wheelchair into Mike's Jeep.

As we pulled onto the long road leading away from the hospital, Mike glances at me. "How did it go?"

"Fine, I guess," I mumbled. "I feel kind of fuzzy. Tired. My head hurts."

I know he wants me to say that I feel *better*. I want to say it too. I want to tell him it worked, that I can already feel the fog lifting. But I can't.

Instead, we drove home in silence, and I hold on to a shred of hope that maybe—just maybe—a miracle will happen.

I had five more treatments to go.

The second treatment came and went. Same routine. Same result. Still not fixed. Still drowning. Still wanting to die every waking moment.

Then came treatment number three.

That's when the lights came back on.

It was like someone flipped a switch in my brain, and for the first time in what felt like forever, there was *peace*. A tiny flicker of hope sparked inside me—like maybe, just maybe, there *was* a way out of the hell I had been living in.

My mom drove me to that treatment. On the way home, I turned to her and asked, "Do you think we could stop at the store? I want to get the ingredients to make chocolate chip cookies."

Not pre-made dough. Not store-bought. I wanted to make them from scratch. *Because I had a taste for them.*

"Of course, honey," she said, her voice thick with emotion.

Looking back, I think she would have driven me straight to the

Tollhouse factory had I asked. For weeks, she had watched me force food down my throat, eating only because I *had* to, because nothing ever sounded good. And now? I *wanted* something. That was huge. That was *everything*.

We didn't talk that day about what my request really meant. But in the years since, she's told me she knew, right then and there, that something inside me had shifted.

Mike noticed it too.

"I knew you were getting better when Amazon packages started showing up at the house again," he told me later.

That might seem small—insignificant, even. But it wasn't.

For so long, I had been incapable of making even the simplest decisions. The idea of shopping, of choosing things *for myself*, had felt impossible.

But now? Now, I was choosing.

And that meant I was *coming back to life*.

At treatment number four, when Dr. Burke asked how my depression symptoms were and if I had noticed any changes, I was finally able to give him a positive answer.

"YES! I think it might be working!" I blurted out, barely restraining myself from throwing my arms around him.

I told him about wanting to bake cookies. How, for the first time in years, I felt a flicker of hope about living and the possibility of overcoming this illness.

The rest of the treatments in the series are harder to recall now, blurred by the memory loss that ECT has left me with. Fortunately, that's the only real side effect I've experienced—one that's common among patients. My memory loss is random, with no pattern or predictability. I've never been able to pinpoint exact time periods that are missing, other than the days immediately before and after a treatment, which always feel fuzzy and impossible to fully remember. Some memories from various points in my life are gone forever, while others can resurface if someone reminds me of the details.

My friends and family have learned to joke about it. If they bring up something and I look at them blankly, they'll laugh and say, *"Oh, that one must have gotten zapped!"* And we move on.

After realizing that memory loss was an unavoidable part of this process, I began taking more detailed notes at work after important conversations. I wanted a record to look back on in case I forgot things—both to clarify details and to ensure I wasn't being misled or manipulated into anything I hadn't agreed to. But ultimately, I consider the memory loss a small price to pay.

Because ECT *worked*.

It gave me my life back.

If losing pieces of my past means I never have to go back to the hell of my depression, then so be it.

I finished the series of treatments, and the next step was maintenance ECT—once every four weeks, with the goal of gradually spacing them out further and further. Maybe one day, I wouldn't need them at all.

My first maintenance treatment was scheduled for mid-December. In the weeks leading up to it, I felt *really* good. No symptoms of depression. I started working again and was managing life independently. Of course, a small, familiar fear lingered in the back of my mind—the *"what if"* whispering that this relief was temporary, that the darkness would creep back in. But for now, I was embracing life again, feeling more like myself than I had in over four years.

For the first time in a long time, I genuinely enjoyed our staff holiday party. I felt an invigorating sense of purpose in leading my team and driving results at work. I was excited to spend Christmas with my friends and family, looking forward to choosing thoughtful gifts for everyone on my list.

I felt *alive* again. At *peace*.

I could think clearly, make decisions, and, most importantly, I could *laugh*—not the forced, hollow kind I had been faking for years, but *real* laughter. I found my quick wit again, cracking jokes and making others laugh, something that had always been a core part of who I was. If you asked anyone to describe me before my depression took hold, that's what they would have said: *Laura is funny.*

And now, finally, I was *me* again.

At my first maintenance ECT appointment, I shared my progress with Dr. Burke.

"I feel great," I told him. "I haven't had any symptoms of depression since my last treatment."

But even as I spoke, I couldn't ignore the internal conflict I had been wrestling with. I had spent so much time reflecting on how difficult this journey had been—how much *shame* and *embarrassment* I still felt about having a mental illness.

I hadn't fully accepted it yet.

I *knew* that what I had was a medical condition—just as real, just as life-threatening if untreated, as diabetes or cancer. But deep down, I was still struggling to come to terms with it. Was this really my reality now?

Mentally ill. Dependent on ECT to feel normal, to function, to survive. I didn't want it to be true.

"Will I have to do this forever?" I finally asked.

Dr. Burke's response was careful, measured, but still unsettling. "Everyone responds differently to treatment, Laura. It's hard to say how long you'll need ECT. But the good news is that it works for you. You have a solution to your depression, and it's available to you for as long as you need it."

He meant it to be reassuring, but all I could hear were the *what ifs* screaming in my mind.

What if I have to do this every four weeks for the rest of my life?
What if, one day, it stops working?
What if, eventually, it erases all of my memories?

There were no answers. Just the same vague reassurance: "Everyone is different." That was when I decided I needed more help. If I was going to accept this diagnosis—if I was going to come to terms with what it meant for my future—I needed someone to help me *process* it.

I needed therapy.

And so, I made the decision to start seeing a therapist—not just to manage my depression, but to help me navigate the overwhelming feelings of uncertainty of living with it. To find a way to *accept* it, once and for all.

Therapy proved to be invaluable in helping me navigate my feelings about mental illness, allowing me to finally accept the reality of what I had experienced. I had been diagnosed with a severe mental illness. At the lowest point of my depression, I had become suicidal and unable to perform even the most basic life functions.

Mental illness is a serious medical condition, one that anyone can develop due to an imbalance in the chemical makeup of their brain. It doesn't discriminate, and—most importantly—it wasn't my fault. I had to accept that managing my mental health would require lifelong diligence—consistent medical care, follow-ups, and treatments to stay well. These were now my truths. I may not have liked them, but I had accepted them.

What I *could not* accept was the stigma surrounding mental illness.

I began to wonder how I could change that.

At one point, it occurred to me how much easier it would have been if I could have simply posted about my struggles on social media—just like people do when they're battling cancer or recovering from surgery. I could have asked for advice, found others who had been through the same thing, and felt less alone.

But that's not how it works with depression.

Because of the stigma surrounding mental health, those of us struggling with it don't feel comfortable sharing our experiences the way we would if the diagnosis had been something more widely accepted—like diabetes or cancer.

There was even a point in my journey when I *wished* I had cancer instead of a mental illness. Because when you have cancer, people *know* what to do. They organize meal trains. They send cards. They call to check in and tell you they're praying for your recovery.

But when you're healing from a *mental* illness?

There's no guidebook for that. No automatic outpouring of support. No casseroles. And it was not necessarily the fault of the people in my circle. It was not my fault. It was *the stigma*.

The stigma tells you that your struggle is embarrassing. Shameful. Ridiculous. It convinces you that if you open up about what you're going through, people will judge you or think you're weak. And how do you even begin to explain the *depth* of suffering when the pain isn't visible?

If someone has never experienced a mental illness—or loved someone who has—they likely won't understand. And taking that risk, the chance of being misunderstood, often feels like a mountain too high to climb.

So we stay silent.

Our struggles become whispers at family gatherings, hushed conversations between friends, never discussed openly. Because people still don't *know* how to respond to mental illness with guaranteed empathy and compassion.

I was one of the lucky ones.

I'm self-employed, and I had an incredible salon manager who could step in and lead my company when I couldn't work. But not everyone has that luxury. Many people don't have the resources or support to take time off. Some even lose their jobs when they disclose that they need time to heal their mental illness. On paper, the symptoms of mental illness can look like poor job performance, laziness, or absenteeism. But it's *not* because the person isn't trying. They are. They're probably fighting like hell.

This period of reflection sparked something in me. In true overachiever fashion, I decided that I was going to single-handedly end the stigma surrounding mental illness *once and for all*.

But how?

I was just one person. A woman in Louisville, Kentucky, trying to take on a centuries-old, worldwide stigma. How was *I* supposed to make a difference?

I quickly realized I couldn't change the entire world overnight. But I *could* start small. I could begin within my own circles—talking about my experience, sharing my story, and creating awareness among the people I already knew. That felt more doable.

So I made a decision.

At our company's kickoff meeting in January 2020, I would tell my staff. Staff meetings had always made me nervous. I poured so much effort into planning them, making sure the content is impactful. And despite leading *hundreds* of meetings throughout my career, this one would be different.

This one would be the most *vulnerable* moment of my life.

Brené Brown would be so proud.

I saved the mental health portion for the very end of the agenda, and as we got closer, I could feel my nerves intensifying.

Here goes nothing, I thought as I took a deep breath and began.

"I know you guys have noticed that there have been periods of time when I'm not at work," I started. "I want to share where I've been, and at the end, I'll explain why I'm telling you all of this."

The room fell silent. All eyes were on me.

I started talking, and suddenly, it was like I was outside of myself, watching the words spill from my mouth.

I told them everything.

How it started. The endless medications, therapies, and treatments I had tried. The details of my ECT treatments—ones I had undergone just weeks before this meeting.

When I finished, I felt two things at once: relief that it was finally *out* and panic about how they would see me now that they *knew*.

To my shock, one of my employees stood up.

She started clapping, tears in her eyes.

"I think it's amazing that you shared this," she said. "And I think you're so brave for going through ECT."

I thanked everyone, humbly wrapped up the meeting, and retreated to my office to collect myself.

The rest of the day, I experienced the *worst* vulnerability hangover of my life.

I worried about what they were thinking. If their perception of me had changed. If they now saw me as weak. If they felt uneasy working for someone with a *mental illness*.

I distracted myself by tackling my to-do list.

Then, suddenly, a text came through.

It was from the brand rep who had attended our meeting that day. And though her message was short, it ignited a fire in me that still burns to this day.

> Laura, I had no idea you struggled with depression. I have struggled with the same thing, and now I don't feel so alone.

Even now, as I write this, those words make me cry.

I had *forgotten* she was even in the meeting—probably because I had been blacking out from the fear of sharing something so deeply personal. But her message connected the dots for me.

This was why it had happened to me.

This was how I was going to use my experience.

If sharing my story could make *one person* feel seen, feel *less alone*, then there was a chance I could also give others the courage to speak up—to ask for help, for themselves or for someone they love.

That day, I was *rewarded* for my courage.

And every time since, whenever I've had the bravery to share my story, the universe—or God—sends me a sign to keep going. A text. A message. A whispered thank-you in passing. Every time, I am reminded that this work *matters*. And so, I press on. That staff meeting was my first experience going public with my mental illness. But at that point, I hadn't even had my first *maintenance* ECT treatment yet.

And, little did I know, in just three short months the entire world would shut down—because of a global pandemic.

Chapter 9

Coming Out of the Mental Illness Closet

By mid-March of 2020, everything had shut down because of COVID-19. I had been able to maintain really good mental health since starting my monthly maintenance ECT treatments, and I was scheduled for my next one at the end of March. But those first few weeks of the shutdown were tough on *everyone*. Like the rest of the world, I was under an extreme amount of stress and uncertainty—especially when it came to my business. There were no clear answers, no guidance on how to proceed.

And here I was, only two and a half months into recovery from a severe mental illness, suddenly thrust into an unprecedented crisis. The weight of what would be required of me—mentally, emotionally—was concerning not just to me, but to everyone who loved me. I tried to stay positive. But as the date for my next ECT treatment approached, I could feel myself *slipping*. I was terrified of what that meant. My mind immediately jumped to worst-case scenarios.

Maybe the ECT isn't going to work now, either.

As if that fear wasn't enough, I had recently learned that Dr. Burke was retiring. My treatments would now be administered by a different psychiatrist—Dr. Spears. I wasn't thrilled about having to adjust to a new doctor, especially when the stakes were this high.

My life *literally* depended on this treatment working. And now I had to put my trust in someone new. I already had sky-high expectations for him.

At my next appointment, when Dr. Spears made his rounds, I told him what was on my mind.

"I'm a little worried that some of my depressive symptoms have returned," I admitted. "I'm feeling overwhelmed, simple decisions are becoming harder, and I'm having negative thoughts."

He nodded and tried to reassure me.

"There's a lot going on in the world right now," he said. "Everyone is feeling a little uneasy. If this treatment doesn't help ease your symptoms, you can come back sooner for additional sessions."

I wanted to believe him. But over the next 24 hours, I *still* wasn't feeling much relief. So I called his office.

"Hi, this is Laura Watkins. I'm an ECT patient of Dr. Spears. I just had a treatment on Monday, and he told me to call if my symptoms didn't improve."

I held my breath, waiting for the receptionist's response.

"Okay, Mrs. Watkins. I'll let him know what's going on and have him get back to you."

I waited. And waited. What was probably *a couple of hours* felt like *months*. My mind spiraled. I had convinced myself that the ECT had stopped working. That I was about to lose my grip on reality again. That I would be facing a massive depressive episode *on top* of trying to keep my business afloat in the middle of a global crisis. It felt impossible.

When my phone finally rang, I picked up immediately, desperation laced in my voice. "What should we do next?" I asked Dr. Spears.

"I think we should do a couple of booster treatments and see if we can get you back to where you were," he suggested. "Let's try two more and see what happens."

At that point, I had nothing to lose.

We scheduled two additional treatments—one on Wednesday and another on Friday—bringing the total to three in the span of a week. And it worked. When I woke up from my nap after the third treatment, I felt *normal* again. I exhaled a *hallelujah* under my breath. The world was still uncertain. I still had mountains to climb. But I knew that if I could maintain my mental health, I could figure the rest out.

In the weeks that followed, things remained unpredictable. But after that series of ECT treatments, as the world slowly adjusted to this new reality, I was able to keep my mental health stable. It took a combination of monthly ECT sessions, medication, and—something I had never prioritized before—self-care.

Before my breakdown, I had always considered self-care to be a *luxury*. A bubble bath. A wine night with friends. Something you did *after* you had pushed yourself to the point of exhaustion. I now knew how *wrong* that mindset was. I had ignored the importance of self-care for so long because I thought it was too indulgent. But in reality, it was *essential*. Through this experience, I learned some of the simplest yet most life-altering lessons—things that, in hindsight, seem so *obvious*, but that I had dismissed for years.

One of the most important? The brain is *just* like any other organ. If you don't take care of it properly, it will get sick. And when it does, it can cause a ripple effect of problems—the worst of which can be suicide.

Our society, especially for women, conditions us to believe that we have to *do it all*—to be everything to everyone, all while smiling and pretending we have it under control. But that's a lie.

Living that way is not sustainable.

Your body and mind will shut down when they've had enough. Mental illness can be caused by so many factors—genetics, unresolved trauma, abuse, tragedy. And if left untreated, the chemicals in your brain can become unbalanced, disrupting your entire mood, personality, and ability to function.

In my case, I truly believe that years of accumulated stress—both *good* and *bad*—without properly caring for my mind led to my treatment-resistant major depressive disorder.

And the irony of *when* it happened?

My most severe symptoms first appeared when my husband retired from the Army. When we finally moved home, closer to family, closer to our village of support. At the time, the very first doctor I saw compared my mental health to a late-crumbling foundation. And now, looking back, I realize how fitting that analogy was.

My brain *waited* until I was home—where I was safest—before it crumbled. Coincidence? I don't think so. My mindset around self-care has completely changed. I no longer think of it as something *nice to have*—a luxury or an indulgence. I see it for what it truly is: a matter of *life and death*.

For me, self-care is now *non-negotiable*.

I once read that we need to rest and recharge with the same intensity that we rise and pursue our endeavors. I couldn't agree more. Now, I *plan* my downtime. I don't over schedule myself. I say no to things more often than I used to.

And guess what? It's *worth it*.

I refuse to compromise my mental health just to fit in or be a part of the action. I rarely experience FOMO anymore. In fact, I joke with some of my peers that we now have JOMO—*the joy of missing out*. I'm no longer impressed by the glorification of busyness that so many people live by. This led me to have another crucial realization about self-care: it's not about what it *is*, but rather what it is *not*. It's *not* just bubble baths and wine nights. It's about creating a personalized self-care *toolkit*—one designed to keep *you* mentally well. And that toolkit will look different for everyone.

At first, my self-care routine consisted of maintenance ECT

treatments, taking both of my prescribed medications daily (along with a Vitamin D supplement), getting at least eight hours of sleep each night, and making sure I scheduled a monthly massage. I also made it a priority to get together with my college girlfriends regularly—because nothing floods my brain with good chemicals like a few hours of uncontrollable laughter.

Over time, I've added to my self-care toolkit as I've discovered new things that bring me joy and enhance my well-being. I share a comprehensive list of these at the end of the book, but the key takeaway is this:

If you don't already have a self-care routine, *start one now*. Because it's not a matter of *if* you'll need it—it's a matter of *when*.

If you take *one* thing away from reading my story, let it be this: self-care is essential to thriving. It allows you to be fully present, accountable, and engaged in the audacious life you deserve. The bottom line? A self-care routine can quite literally save your life.

As I moved further into recovery, I was able to space out my maintenance ECT treatments by four weeks at a time. By 2022—nearly three years after my first series of treatments in 2019—I had reached a point where I could comfortably go 12 weeks between treatments. But every time I tried to push past that 12-week mark, I felt myself slipping. I would inevitably need another treatment to get back to feeling *well* again.

At first, I struggled with this reality. I still blamed myself when I couldn't go longer between treatments, as if it were some kind of *personal failure*. So I made a decision: I wouldn't try to extend beyond 12 weeks anymore—not until I was *truly* ready. Instead of feeling disappointed in myself for not making it to 16 weeks, I chose to focus on what was *working*.

Still, I knew I had some lingering feelings to process.

So, I returned to talk therapy—yet another tool in my self-care toolkit. I needed to work through my acceptance of *needing* ECT treatments, no matter how much I wished I didn't. And because I wanted to make sure I was covering *every* possible factor in my recovery, I also decided to work with a functional medicine nurse. I wanted to explore what other changes—through diet, supplements, or lifestyle—could support my mental health.

Thankfully, I had already taken the GeneSight test, which identifies how your unique genetic makeup affects your body's response to different medications and supplements. With that information in hand, my functional medicine nurse began educating me about the biological mechanisms that could be contributing to my depression.

For example—she shared that 90-95% of serotonin (one of the key chemicals that regulates mood) is actually produced in the gut. Not the brain. The gut. In fact, there are *trillions* of microbes in the gut that produce chemicals affecting how the brain functions. That means gut health is directly tied to mental health. This was a *huge* lightbulb moment for me. The first supplement my functional nutritionist recommended? A probiotic—to support a healthier gut microbiome.

Next, she explained the importance of Omega-3 fatty acids for brain health. These are found in oily fish like salmon, which I now eat more often, but I also take an Omega-3 supplement to ensure I'm getting enough.

Then, we spent time discussing inflammation and how it contributes to conditions like Major Depressive Disorder. It turns out that chronic inflammation can disrupt the brain's ability to regulate mood, and decreasing inflammation can play a key role in improving mental health.

We also talked a *lot* about poop. Apparently, I wasn't eliminating waste often enough. Proper detoxification is crucial for decreasing inflammation in the body. My nurse explained that if toxins aren't removed efficiently, they build up and wreak havoc—including on mental health. To help with this, she added Magnesium to my supplement regimen. This not only regulates digestion but also plays a role in relaxation and stress reduction.

I know—TMI.

But trust me, it *matters*.

By the end of my six weeks of coaching, my list of supplements had grown significantly. Here's what I take now:

Prescribed Medications:

- Effexor (Venlafaxine) – for depression & anxiety
- Remeron (Mirtazapine) – for depression & sleep

Vitamins and Supplements:

- Vitamin D – supports mood & immune function
- Methylfolate – supports brain function & energy
- Probiotic – for gut health (linked to serotonin production)
- Omega-3 – supports brain function & reduces inflammation
- Magnesium – supports digestion, relaxation, and sleep
- NAC (N-Acetyl Cysteine) – replenishes antioxidants & nourishes the brain
- Berberine – linked to improved brain health

Each of these plays a role in supporting my overall well-being. By combining ECT, medication, therapy, self-care, and a tailored supplement plan, I have finally found a system that works for *me*. And that's the key: finding what works for you. Recovery isn't about finding a one-size-fits-all solution. It's about uncovering what *your* body, *your* brain, and *your* soul need to *thrive*. For me, it's been a combination of science, self-awareness, and self-compassion.

I'll always be evolving, learning, and fine-tuning my approach to wellness. But one thing I know for sure? Self-care isn't optional. It's *essential*.

In my quest to uncover every possible solution for managing my depression, I started identifying other areas of my life where I could make changes that would positively impact my mental health. One of the most eye-opening moments came from my close friend Samantha. During COVID, she went alcohol-free and wrote a book, Alive AF: One Mom's Journey to Becoming Alcohol Free, about her experience healing from crippling anxiety—how it had been fueled by her drinking.

Through Samantha, I started learning more about alcohol. I found out how it's processed by the body, how it affects the brain, and how we are influenced from an early age to accept drinking as normal, despite its well-documented effects on our health. I had never really thought about it before. At the very least, alcohol is classified as a depressant, and that fact alone was enough to convince me to limit my consumption to *almost never* these days.

That wasn't the only habit I started questioning.

I have always been a sucker for a McDonald's fountain Diet Coke. My love for diet soda started in my teenage years, thanks to my parents' fascination with Tab (a popular diet drink in the '80s). Since then, I had been drinking large amounts of diet soda every day. So, imagine my disappointment when, during my deep dive into mental health research, I stumbled upon an article stating that people who regularly drink diet sodas are 30% more likely to develop depression—and that artificial sweeteners also contribute to inflammation.

Well, shit.

No more alcohol. No more Diet Coke. And on top of that, I now had so many prescribed medications and supplements that I had to carry around a pill organizer the size of something my grandfather with Parkinson's used to have in his suitcase.

What kind of fresh hell is this?

At first, I resisted. But when I weighed my options, the choice was clear: I could either continue consuming things that I now *knew* were negatively impacting my brain, or I could prioritize my mental health and live well. And when I considered the alternative—the deep, dark hole of depression that made me want to die—it didn't even feel like a sacrifice. It was a lifeline.

Now that I was months—even years—into my recovery, I found myself reflecting more and more on how sick I had been. How dangerously close I had come to ending my own life. And I started wondering...

Did I have the courage to go public with my experience?

For a while, I went back and forth. But eventually, I realized something: If sharing my story could help even one person—if it could encourage someone to seek help or remind them they weren't alone—then it was worth the risk.

Of course, the *what ifs* immediately crept in:

What if people think I'm crazy?

What if I'm accused of oversharing?

What if I lose credibility with my team or colleagues in the beauty industry?

What if I embarrass my family by sharing that they are related to a "mentally ill" person?

What if people are mean in the comments?

What if I get canceled?

But then I flipped the script:

What if someone reads my story and feels less alone?

What if my post helps break the stigma surrounding mental health?

What if someone I know is struggling in silence because they are too ashamed to ask for help?

What if... What if... What if...

Finally, in July of 2021, I did it. I hit "publish" on my first public social media post about my mental health.

"If you're like I used to be, you probably think mental illness is something that only affects "crazy people" or, at the very least, people who have experienced extreme trauma.

But what if I told you it can happen to the mom you see at school pickup? Or the fun, social, "life of the party" friend with the infectious laugh? Or the woman who owns a small business down the street, sells Aveda, and gives a mean blowout? Or the woman with a loving, supportive family, an amazing husband, and no history of trauma? The truth is, mental illness can happen to anyone. Anywhere. At any time.

I know this because it happened to me.

I was first diagnosed with Major Depressive Disorder in 2015 when I fell into a depressive episode that hit me out of nowhere. I've battled severe depression on and off ever since. I've tried multiple therapies, medications, and even Electroconvulsive Therapy (ECT).

At first, I was ashamed. I kept asking myself, What do you even have to be depressed about? But here's what I've learned: The brain is an organ, just like the heart, the liver, or the pancreas. And just like any other organ, it can get sick.

We don't shame people for getting treatment for heart disease, diabetes, or cancer.

So why do we still hold so much stigma around mental illness? I'm ready to do my part to change that stigma. And with your help, we can make a difference. What do you say we start talking more about it?"

As soon as I hit "post," I immediately felt like I was going to vomit. And then came the waiting.

I kept refreshing my screen to see if anyone had seen it yet, liked it, or responded. My heart pounded as the notifications started rolling in. To my *huge* relief, none of my worst fears came true. In fact, it was the opposite. So many people liked the post. Several left positive comments, thanking me for sharing or reinforcing what I had said about mental health.

But what really shocked me?

The *private messages.*

People I never would have expected reached out to me, sharing their own struggles with mental illness. They told me they had been suffering in silence and that my post made them feel safe enough to open up. I had no idea so many people were going through the same thing. And I never would have known—if I hadn't shared my own story first.

At the end of 2021, my sister-in-law, Joann, suggested we try a bootcamp-style exercise class together. I had seen the classes advertised and even knew a few people who attended. But I always assumed it would be way too intense for me. There was no way in *hell* I would have had the nerve to go alone. But I knew regular exercise would be another valuable tool in my self-care toolkit. And now that I had a friend to go with, maybe I'd give it a try.

It was just as hard as I expected. The coaches were great, but I had to modify a *lot* of the exercises just to make it through. We set a goal to attend the 6:30 am class three days a week. For the most part, we've stuck to it. The workouts never get easier, but I've gotten stronger. On the days I go, I have more energy and better focus. And, of course, exercise floods the brain with endorphins, which help improve mood—something I desperately needed.

Now that my mental health is stabilized with medication and ECT, I have the capacity to commit to regular exercise. But when I was in the depths of my depression, it felt impossible. Even though I *knew* exercise would help, I could barely function. The thought of working out felt overwhelming, and my negative thought patterns convinced me it wouldn't make a difference anyway.

Now, these bootcamp classes are another non-negotiable in my self-care routine. And even though I hate every minute of it, I always feel better when it's done.

By January of 2023, I was feeling great. No symptoms of depression. For the previous year, I had been faithfully showing up for my

ECT treatments every 12 weeks, afraid that if I pushed past that window, I would start to slip again—as had always been the case.

The treatment itself went as usual. But this time, something felt...off. For the next few days, I struggled to bounce back like I normally did. I felt stuck in a funk—more tired than usual, lacking energy, just *off*. The symptoms weren't severe, and I wasn't even sure I could call them depression, but I was afraid they could be a sign of something bad.

I called Dr. Spears. When we finally spoke, I explained my concerns.

"It took me a few days to feel normal after this treatment," I told him. "Usually, I come home, take a nap, and when I wake up, I feel pretty good and get back to my normal routine. This time, it took a couple of days. Is it possible that because I went into this treatment already feeling great, the ECT actually took me backwards a bit?"

"I don't think so," he said. "This was probably just a fluke. But if you're open to it, let's see how you're feeling at 10 weeks instead of 12. If you're still feeling great, let's push the next treatment out a couple more weeks and see what happens. In some cases, patients eventually reach a point where they don't need treatments at all. We'll have to wait and see."

I hesitated. "Alright, I guess we can do that," I agreed reluctantly. "But how quickly can I get in if I feel myself slipping again?"

He assured me that if I needed a treatment, I could get in within a day or two. So we decided to wait and see—even though I hated that approach. For years, *waiting and seeing* had never worked out in my favor. It had always led to a downward spiral until I had found ECT.

I wanted to scream: *Wait and see my ass! I've waited and I've seen, and it hasn't worked out so well for me.*

But what other choice did I have?

As week 10 approached, I still felt great—no symptoms of depression. At week 12, still nothing. So we rescheduled for 16 weeks and agreed that if anything changed, I could call immediately. I kept waiting for the shift. Any day now, I told myself, I would feel *off*—that familiar fog would roll in, and I'd need to get in ASAP for a treatment.

But in the meantime, I stayed diligent about self-care, checking in with myself daily. I monitored my mood, my energy levels, my thoughts—looking for any tiny sign of a depressive episode creeping in. At 16 weeks, still nothing. So we pushed to 20 weeks. I almost couldn't believe it.

I had *resigned* myself to the idea that ECT would always be a part of my life. Even though Dr. Spears had reassured me—*multiple times*—that ECT would never "fry my brain to the point where I couldn't remember anything," I still wasn't entirely convinced. I went ahead and completed my yearly labs and EKG—both of which are required annually for ECT patients. I also extended my referral with my insurance company to cover me through June, since my last treatment in January marked the end of my most recent approval. I wanted to be ready—prepared to go back for treatment the *moment* I felt myself slipping.

Because I *knew* this couldn't last.

But it did. At 24 weeks (6 months!), I still felt great. No depressive symptoms. No fog. No spiral. I kept waiting. Kept *seeing*. Kept pushing out my next treatment another four weeks. And still, I felt mentally well. Could it be that—just maybe—I had *beat* this? In addition to ECT, I had made several other key lifestyle changes that I believe played a significant role in my long-term recovery.

I dove deep into functional medicine, exploring how supplements, gut health, and vitamin deficiencies contribute to mental health.

Here's what I learned:

1. Vitamin D Deficiency & Mental Health

Vitamin D is critical for mood regulation. I discovered that many people—myself included—are severely deficient. Supplementing with Vitamin D became an essential part of my regimen.

2. Gut Health & The Brain

Since 90-95% of serotonin—the neurotransmitter that regulates mood—is actually produced in the gut, not the brain, the gut and brain are directly connected. If your gut isn't functioning properly, your mental health can suffer. (Reference: <u>Healthline – Gut-Brain Connection</u>) To improve gut health, I started taking a probiotic and focused on reducing inflammation through diet and supplements.

3. MTHFR Gene Mutation & Depression

I learned that I have an MTHFR gene mutation, which affects my body's ability to convert folic acid into its active form (methylfolate). This genetic mutation is linked to higher rates of depression and anxiety. Once I started supplementing with Methylfolate, I noticed a difference in my energy levels and mood stability. (Reference: <u>MTHFR Gene Info – Healthline</u>)

4. NAC & Reducing Inflammation

Inflammation plays a huge role in Major Depressive Disorder. I started taking NAC (N-Acetyl Cysteine), which helps reduce oxidative stress and supports brain health. (Reference: <u>NAC Benefits – Healthline</u>)

I never thought I would be able to go six months—or longer—without an ECT treatment. For years, it felt like the only thing keeping me alive. But here I am, still waiting and seeing, still getting further and further away from my last treatment—and still feeling well. I don't know what the future holds. I don't know if I'll ever need ECT again.

But for now, I know this:

- Functional medicine, supplements, and understanding my body have made a profound difference in my mental health.

- Self-care is non-negotiable.
- And there is always hope—even when you think you've tried everything.

I may not have all the answers, but I finally believe in the possibility that I have found true healing.

And maybe—just maybe—I've beaten this for good.

Chapter 10

The Awakening

I knew as soon as I saw the text that bad news was coming.

I make it a regular practice to schedule one-on-one meetings outside the salon with my staff—whether it's grabbing coffee or going to lunch for those who are interested. Even though I've scaled back the number of hours I spend in the salon each week, I still believe it's important to have regular touch points with my team. These moments reassure them that I'm invested in their growth, and they give me an opportunity to get to know them on a personal level. It's also a chance for them to voice concerns, share frustrations, or talk about their career goals.

I love this part of my job. Coaching and mentoring young adults as they begin their journey in the industry is incredibly fulfilling. Watching them evolve into the best versions of themselves brings me so much joy. Even though these meetings require a significant investment of my time and energy, they always pay off. They allow me to keep a pulse on the team's dynamics and the individual aspirations of each stylist.

Stephanie and I had plans to meet for lunch on Thursday, so when her text came through on Sunday asking,

> Can we change our lunch catch-up to my lunch hour on Tuesday?

I knew something was off.
A knot formed in my stomach.
I decided to test the waters a bit with my response:

> Did you need to talk to me sooner? Something on your mind?

That exchange happened around 4 p.m. When I still hadn't heard back, I sent a follow-up message:

> Girl! Leaving me hanging?

Her response came quickly:

> Sorry, I've just had a lot on my mind and didn't know exactly how to approach you with it.

Great. Here we go again.
I took a deep breath and replied.

> I can meet you for coffee at 9 a.m. tomorrow.

I arrived early for our coffee date and went ahead and ordered for both of us. As soon as she sat down, I went straight to the point.

"So, lay it on me," I said.

Stephanie exhaled. "Well, I wanted to tell you that I just signed a lease on a salon suite this morning. I'd like for this to be my two weeks notice, if that's okay with you."

Are you freaking kidding me?

That's what I wanted to say. Instead, I remained calm, even as my mind started racing.

Why does it always happen like this?

Why do they always make these big decisions so quickly—without even asking for my advice or support?

In all my years as a salon owner, I have never raised my voice at an employee. I pride myself on being a leader who leads with heart—someone who connects with my team and constantly reminds them how much I care. I support them, whether they choose to work for me or move on to new opportunities.

So why, in these moments, do they treat me as the enemy?

Why do they suddenly feel like they can't trust me with the truth?

I genuinely care about everyone who works for me.

I make it a priority to know them personally—their goals, dreams, and struggles. My manager and I meet with them regularly to provide feedback and identify areas for growth. If they want to specialize in a particular skill, we find the right education, help fund the cost, and even pay them for their time in class.

I celebrate their wins.

Personal text messages, shout-outs in our group chat, recognition at team meetings, handwritten cards, thoughtful gifts—I make sure they feel valued. Every birthday and work anniversary is acknowledged with their favorite treats, flowers, and a bonus for each year they've been with me.

I check in on them when they're sick.

I offer benefits like paid time off, telehealth access, and ten free therapy sessions per year with a licensed therapist.

I answer texts and calls after hours and follow through on every commitment I make to them. I often see more potential in my team members than they see in themselves, and I work tirelessly to build their confidence. More than just a boss, I am a mentor, a life coach, and sometimes even a therapist. They share personal details with me that people my age would have never shared with an employer. And I welcome it—because that's the kind of leader I choose to be.

And yet, in moments like this, it feels like none of that matters.

Rarely do I receive a thank you or even the slightest acknowledgment for everything I do. Most of the time, I don't let it get to me—after all, I choose to lead this way. But when they leave, I just wish they would consider me a mentor in the same way they counted on me for everything else while they were here. Why in the world wouldn't they ask for my guidance when making such a critical decision in their careers? At the very least, why wouldn't they take me up on my offer to help set them up for success? Why don't they see that going independent is about so much more than just doing hair?

When a stylist decides they want to work for themselves, they have two primary options. The first is to rent a chair in an existing salon that offers booth rentals. The second is to rent a suite, a newer business model in the beauty industry that allows stylists to lease a small, private room within a larger building designed for beauty professionals. This suite setup feels like a mini salon of their own—equipped with a chair, hair station, and shampoo bowl.

In both cases, they are now responsible for:
- ✔ Paying weekly rent
- ✔ Supplying all of their products, tools, and equipment
- ✔ Handling marketing and branding
- ✔ Booking every client appointment
- ✔ Filing and paying their own taxes

And that's just the beginning. What they usually fail to consider is the sheer number of extra hours they'll have to work beyond their time behind the chair.

It's no longer just about cutting and coloring hair—it's also about:

- Responding to messages and calls to book appointments

- Managing inventory and purchasing supplies
- Making supply runs to restock products
- Creating content for marketing their services
- Finding and retaining clients

Going independent means they aren't just hairstylists anymore. They are business owners. And being great at doing hair isn't enough. To make it sustainable, they need business knowledge and financial literacy—something many of them don't realize until they're drowning in unexpected responsibilities.

Every salon owner in this industry has seen this story play out time and time again. Stylists come to work for me right out of cosmetology school because they see the value in what I provide. I invest over $10,000 in training, mentorship, and support to set them up for success behind the chair. I teach them everything they need to know—not just about hair but about client retention, consultation skills, business etiquette, and industry growth. And if that wasn't enough? I fill their books for them. I bring them clients and provide opportunities most salon owners wouldn't even consider offering.

And yet...after all that?

Most of them still don't have the respect to be honest with me when they decide they want to leave. Instead, they make decisions in secret, moving forward with no conversation, no warning, and no acknowledgment of everything I've done for them. I am so sick of it. I can't help but wonder—why?

Once they become successful working for me, why do they suddenly feel the need to go out on their own? Do they really believe they did it all on their own? Are they blind to the fact that their success was a team effort—a combination of their hard work and the unwavering support of a leadership team, a structured business, and a strong salon brand that I built for them? Do they not see the mentorship, guidance, and investment I poured into them every step of the way?

As I sat across from Stephanie, the next thought that hit me was —*who else is going with her?*

I took a deep breath and asked, "Does anyone else on the staff know you're leaving?"

Stephanie hesitated. "Well...Jessica knows because we're doing a suite together."

Are you freaking kidding me?!

I felt my face heat up, but I managed to keep my voice controlled —just barely.

"Well, that's nice," I said, my tone laced with more sarcasm than I intended. "Does she plan on telling me?"

Stephanie nodded. "Yes. She's just really scared to have the conversation with you...but she's planning on it."

Scared? To have a conversation with me?

Give me a break.

This is the same Jessica who has sat in my office on multiple occasions, confiding in me about her personal struggles. We shared many deep conversations—and she's too scared to tell me about a career move? I clenched my jaw. It was beyond frustrating.

I continued my conversation with Stephanie and quickly realized that two weeks probably wasn't a realistic amount of time for her to keep working while keeping her plans confidential, which is a requirement I have in these situations. I made this rule because it's just too awkward and uncomfortable for the guests. If they want to follow their stylist, they often feel afraid to say so, worried they'll offend the salon. If they want to stay, they don't want to tell the stylist directly, especially while sitting in their chair mid-service. It creates tension, not just for them, but for the entire salon.

The longer a stylist stays after they've mentally and emotionally checked out, the worse it is for the culture of the business. It's not fair to the team that remains, still committed and working hard. When I asked Stephanie if she thought she could keep things confidential for the full two weeks, she hesitated. She knew it would be too long and asked if I would consider letting her leave after one week instead. I told her I'd need the day to think about it.

I decided to consult my leadership team before making a final decision. There was still a lot to process, and I had several hours of work ahead of me. I tried to focus, but the uneasy feeling in my stomach wouldn't go away. I took note of it, remembering the last time I felt this way—when we had a significant turnover at the salon a couple of years ago. I prayed this wasn't the beginning of another downward spiral.

It had been a while since I'd lost stylists like this. The ones who had left recently had done so for other reasons—life changes, moves, terminations—but not to go independent. This was the first time that I was dealing with this situation again since my last experience with severe depression. The last time it happened, I lost multiple staff members in a short period, and it pushed me into a dark place I couldn't pull myself out of. I was terrified of falling back into that.

This is where the story is different than any of the other times I'd been faced with turnover. Instead of giving in to panic and the inevitable downward spiral it would cause, I intentionally leaned into self-care and the routines I'd worked so hard to establish for myself. After finishing the tasks on my list, I decided to head home and go for a walk. The sun was shining, and the fresh air would help clear my head. Maybe it would give me some perspective. When I got back, my husband was home from work. I sat down with him and told him everything. I needed his advice, even though I already had a feeling what he was going to say.

"You have to go ahead and cut them loose," he said. "They've already mentally quit. Keeping them there for another week will just give them more time to talk about it with the staff and guests.

That's not going to work. You've been through this before, and you know I'm right."

Damn. I hated when he was right.

That evening, I let Stephanie and Jessica know they wouldn't be returning to finish out the two weeks notice. They weren't happy with me, but I kept telling myself this was the right decision. It had to be. Now, I had my next hurdle to face—breaking the news to the rest of the staff. That meant I had to go in and lead the morning huddle, something I didn't usually do anymore. I posted a message in our team group, asking everyone to arrive a few minutes early so I could make an announcement. I knew that would immediately set off a flurry of messages behind the scenes. The rumor mill was already spinning.

But this wasn't something I could delegate to my leaders. It wouldn't be fair to them, and what kind of message would it send if I pushed my responsibility onto someone else? Some things just have to come from the top. This is the part of business ownership that no one talks about. There are moments where you have to step in and do things you don't want to do—because no one else can. And those moments? They're lonely. When the responsibility falls squarely on your shoulders to say the right thing, do the right thing, and handle it all with professionalism and grace, it takes guts. It takes determination. And, quite frankly, it's exhausting.

There are days when I just want to throw in the towel.

The emotional strength and resilience it takes to be a leader can be absolutely crushing. If you don't set yourself up for success with a solid self-care plan, a therapist when you need one, and the ability to detach emotionally when the situation calls for it, your job will destroy you.

That night, I cooked a nutritious meal for my family, sat down with them to eat, and decided to read for a bit before taking my medication and heading to bed. It was my way of winding down, trying to keep my mind from spinning too much before morning. I woke up after a solid eight hours of sleep, but the moment I opened my eyes, the nerves hit me. Today was the team huddle, and I was about to stand in front of my staff and deliver news that I knew would be met with mixed reactions.

But first, I had a bootcamp class with my sister-in-law, our regular morning workout. I had no excuse to skip it. So I got into my workout clothes, left the house, and pushed my body to its limits for an hour. It helped, but the weight in my chest remained. When I got back home, I wrote out my talking points, took a deep breath, and got dressed. Then, I headed out with my daughter for the school drop-off. I must have practiced my speech at least 50 times during the drive, running through every possible way it could go.

As I pulled into the parking lot and stepped out of the car, my heart was racing.

"Okay, guys...I know you aren't used to seeing me here for huddles in the morning, and I'm sure many of you already know what I'm about to say," I started.

A few people shifted in their seats, but no one looked up.

"Stephanie and Jessica let me know that they signed a lease yesterday and are going into business together in a suite."

Silence. Heads down.

You could have heard a pin drop in the break room.

"In the last fifteen years of owning a business, I've had probably 20 to 30 employees leave. And if I've learned anything from those experiences, it's that the longer someone continues working after they've already mentally and emotionally quit, the worse it turns out. So I've decided that yesterday was their last day working here, and they won't be back."

Still no eye contact. Still heads down.

"These are never easy decisions to make, but my priority has to be for our team's culture and for the people who are still here—who believe in me and our mission."

A couple of pairs of eyes lifted. A few small nods.

"We work in an industry with a tremendous amount of heart, and I know emotions will be running high in the next few days. You may be frustrated with me for this decision, and things may feel a little messy for a while. But with change comes opportunity. Many of you who have had white space on your books are about to get busier and start making more money."

Did I see a glimmer of hope? Maybe even a smile or two?

"I'm here and available if you have questions or want to talk about this further. And I think it would be great if we plan a happy hour later this week to say goodbye to Stephanie and Jessica and wish them well in their new venture."

Several nods. More eye contact.

"All right, you guys, have a great day. I'm here if you need me."

With that, I left the huddle and escaped to my office, closing the door behind me. I took a deep breath and let it out. I did it. I said what I needed to say, with confidence, without too much shakiness in my voice. My heart was still pounding, and I felt a little light-headed, but at least that part was over. Now I could start preparing for the fallout.

I opened my email, forcing myself to focus on something mundane. I made a mental note of the staff members who hadn't been at huddle and would need to hear the same message from me personally. I didn't want anyone learning about this through whispers in the break room. They deserved to hear it from me.

I glanced at the clock. My writer's group Zoom meeting was about to start.

For a second, I considered skipping it. I had too much going on. My mind was spinning. But then I reminded myself—this group was something I had committed to. This was one of my personal priorities for the year, and I wasn't going to let stress pull me away from the things that were important to me.

It never fails. Whenever I try to talk myself out of something I

Something Feels Off

know I should be doing—like this meeting—I end up getting the exact message I need to hear.

Today was no different.

Samantha, our group leader, started by asking everyone how their writing was going and what we were working on. When it was my turn, I admitted that I hadn't been doing much writing in the last week. Instead, I found myself talking about what had been going on at work.

Without even realizing it, I started saying things like, "This is just part of the business. It's been a while since I've lost stylists, but so far, I'm managing things pretty well. I've gotten great sleep despite losing team members, which a few years ago would have sent me into a spiral…"

Samantha interrupted me. "This. This is exactly what you need to be writing about."

And then it hit me.

Holy shit! I had done the work.

I was mentally well. I was navigating a difficult situation with clarity and strength. A few years ago, losing stylists like this would have wrecked me. It would have sent me into a deep depression, questioning everything, struggling to function.

But now?

I had put in the work—the countless hours of therapy, the multiple ECT treatments, the follow-ups with my psychiatrist, the endless medication trials, and the commitment to taking my medication and supplements every single day. I had prioritized self-care—over 200 bootcamp workouts, drinking 100 ounces of water a day, living (mostly) alcohol-free (Diet Coke is a harder battle), walking miles to clear my head, carving out intentional time to laugh with girlfriends, seeking guidance from mentors, choosing to care for myself, even when I didn't feel like it.

The massages I book, even when I'm tempted to cancel because I feel too busy. The meditations. The endless search for new ways to take care of my brain. The unwavering expectation I have for myself to get eight good hours of sleep. The willingness to let go of what no longer serves me.

All of it.

Every struggle. Every tear. Every moment I wanted to give up but didn't. This was the reward. Maybe it was God. Maybe it was the universe. Maybe it was just years of persistence finally paying off. Whatever it was, I saw it for what it was—a victory.

The very thing that once would have broken me was now something I could handle with strength, grace, and gratitude. I used to think my greatest achievement would be some big milestone in my business. Some external win that would prove I had finally made it. But now I realized...this was it. Not a number on a financial statement. Not a prestigious award. Not external validation. It was this moment. Right here. Right now. The realization that I did it.

I was healthy.

I was strong.

And nothing—not even losing stylists, not even the uncertainty of what was ahead—could take that away from me. I sat there for a moment, letting the realization sink in.

This wasn't just about losing employees. It wasn't about business decisions or revenue projections or the challenges of leadership. This was about me. About how far I had come. About the fact that I was sitting here, processing a difficult situation—not crumbling under the weight of it.

A few years ago, I would have been spiraling. I would have let the self-doubt creep in, questioning whether I was a good leader, whether I was failing, whether I was even capable of continuing. I would have been crushed under the pressure, drowning in anxiety, losing sleep, searching for an escape from the heaviness of it all.

But now?

Now, I was clear-headed. Now, I could navigate this. That wasn't by accident. That wasn't luck. That was years of work—the kind of work that no one else sees, the kind that happens in the quiet moments, when no one is watching. I closed my laptop after the writer's group ended and sat still for a moment, staring at the wall of my office. I knew there was more to do. More conversations to have. More planning to ensure the business kept running smoothly despite the changes.

But for that moment, I let myself feel the win.

For the first time in my life and because of the priority I have intentionally applied to my own mental health and self-care, I was finally at a stable place. Where, by taking care of myself, I was able to take care of the collective mental health of my team. I made a decision about the salon that I knew was right for all of us.

It wasn't the kind of victory that comes with a celebration, with confetti and applause. It was quieter than that. More personal. It was the victory of resilience. The victory of becoming the person I had fought so hard to be.

I picked up my phone and saw a message from one of my team members.

> Hey, I just wanted to say I know today wasn't easy for you, and I appreciate you. I'm excited to step up and take on more clients. I believe in this place. I believe in you.

I smiled.

This was why I kept going. Because for every person who left, there were still people who stayed. People who believed in what we were building, who saw the value in being part of something bigger than themselves.

And me?

I wasn't just surviving anymore. I was thriving. I grabbed my bag, took one last deep breath, and stepped out of my office.

It was time to get back to work.

A goal of mine has always been to hit $1 million in sales, and I've been chasing that goal since 2008, when I first opened my salon. I always thought that would be the pinnacle of success for me and my business. At times, I've come close, but I've never quite hit it. Whether it was staff turnover or a global pandemic, something always seemed to stand in the way of this ultimate sales goal—this number I believed would prove my worth and finally make me feel as if I had *arrived* at success.

Now, I find myself wondering why I placed so much importance on that number. Why was I so focused on the destination instead of celebrating all the achievements along the way?

Don't get me wrong, I would be incredibly proud to say that I—just a girl from Bullitt County, the one whose potential her own teachers and principal dismissed—built a team that generated $1 million in sales from a 1,600-square-foot salon. If I could hit $1 million, maybe *Business First*, a local business publication, would finally do a story on me—something I've been hoping for, especially since they told me when I first opened that a salon opening in Louisville "wasn't newsworthy."

If I could just hit that $1 million.

Maybe someday I will. Maybe I won't.

But now, I see the bigger picture so much more clearly.

My team and I have done the work. We've built sustainable systems to keep the business running. We've prepared for the valleys, ensuring that when challenges come—and they always do—we're ready. Because of those systems, I had enough cash flow to weather the loss of stylists. And with two new stylists in our training program, in just a couple of months, we'd start replacing that lost revenue.

There will always be unknowns as a business owner. Each of us defines success differently. Along the way, there will be things we can't control and others we wish we could change or let go.

But I'll tell you this—the feeling I had when it all came into focus, when I finally *understood*—that was worth more than any financial milestone I could have imagined.

I realized that the personal work I had done—the fight to escape death, the years of healing, the preparation and discipline it took to arrive at a place where I am mentally strong, confident, and at peace despite the chaos around me at my salon—that was the pinnacle of success.

And I had achieved it.

Chapter 11

Let's Change the Conversation

Mental illness took four years of my life away. It convinced me that killing myself would be a better option than living with Major Depressive Disorder. It is an experience I wouldn't wish on my worst enemy. In the darkest days of my depression I would ask myself:

Why is this happening to me?

What have I done to deserve this?

Why am I being punished in this way?

I had numerous conversations with God pleading with him to make me well. In my most desperate times I even began to bargain with him. *If you make me well, I promise I will spend the rest of my life trying to be a beacon of light for others who are suffering in this way.*

In 2014, the year before I was diagnosed with Major Depressive Disorder, I attended Oprah Winfrey's 'The Life You Want Weekend Experience' in Houston, Texas. I met a friend and fellow salon owner there who shared my love for all things Oprah and we made a weekend out of it. This electrifying event included two days of learning and being inspired by Oprah and some of her friends— Deepok Chopra, Rob Bell, Elizabeth Gilbert, and Ilanya Vanzant. It was one of the most inspiring experiences I've ever been to and there were a couple of nuggets that especially resonated with me from the weekend.

The first was that everybody has a calling and it is our job in life to pay attention to that calling.

The second was that many of the things that happen to us have also happened for us and in those moments we get to choose how we want to respond. These seemed like profound learnings at the time and I grabbed onto them even though I wasn't convinced I'd found my calling yet or had much time to reflect on the major things that had happened to me and see them as happening for me.

None of these teachings would hit their exact mark until 2020 when I finally saw a light at the end of the deep, dark tunnel I had been in. Then, I decided to make good on my promise to become that light for others struggling with mental health. I had the opportunity to take something that happened to me and turn it into something that I can do to lift others up. So I began to think of ways I could integrate mental health awareness into my role as a business owner and industry leader to start.

There is a lot of discussion in the salon industry about the disruption Gen Z is bringing to what we—Gen X, Boomers, and maybe some Millennials—thought was the standard way of doing business. These "kids" are often labeled as lazy, irresponsible, and unwilling to work, among other criticisms. I'll admit, I do sometimes get frustrated with their naïve thinking and the bold demands they make of us as leaders—demands I never would have had the nerve to make of my supervisors.

However, one of the things the younger generations are absolutely getting right is their approach to mental health and their insistence on work-life balance. Unlike previous generations, they are not afraid to talk about mental health, and in doing so, they have created much more awareness around it.

Unfortunately, this awareness likely stems from personal experience. According to the National Alliance on Mental Illness (NAMI), one in three adolescents aged 18-25 experiences a mental illness each year, and suicide is the third leading cause of death in this same age group. With unlimited access to information and technology, along with the relentless pressures of social media, it's no wonder adolescents today are experiencing anxiety and depression at alarming rates—far earlier than people in my generation ever did.

I was in my forties before I experienced mental illness or even became aware of what mental health really was. In today's world, that's considered *late*.

I was raised by Boomers who didn't talk about mental health, nor did they really understand it. My parents were loving and nurturing, but we weren't given much knowledge about our mental well-being, what it meant, or how to take care of it. That kind of learning came later—when I had to learn it. I don't blame them for that; it's just the way it was.

Looking back, I'm sure there were kids in my high school struggling with anxiety and depression, but we didn't hear about it. Instead, they were probably labeled as lazy, unmotivated, or even "crazy." We used to joke about stress, saying things like, *If this gets any worse, they'll have to commit me to Our Lady of Peace*—a well-known mental hospital in Louisville. That's how ignorant I was about mental health. I assumed everyone in that hospital was either crazy, weak, incapable of handling life, or suffering from some unimaginable trauma they couldn't overcome.

I thought that when you felt uneasy, you simply acknowledged it and *powered through* until it eventually went away.

Not a sustainable strategy, as I later found out.

Gen Z, on the other hand, is deeply aware of mental health and openly comfortable discussing it. Not to say that some people don't take advantage of the conversation—because yes, there are always those who misuse it as an excuse—but I believe that the majority of people who claim to struggle with mental health genuinely do. If we, as leaders, can create a safe space for them to be honest about their struggles, we have a powerful opportunity—not only to support them through it but also to retain them on our teams.

Despite the progress that has been made, the stigma surrounding mental health remains strong. Many people are still too uncomfortable to have a vulnerable conversation with their boss about what they're experiencing, even though they wouldn't hesitate to share a physical illness.

Think about it. If an employee came to us and said, "I have the flu, and I need a couple of days to rest and recover." would we question them? Would we judge them? Of course not.

So why is it any different if they come to us and say, "I've been experiencing severe anxiety, and I had a panic attack on my way to work this morning. I need to take a couple of days to check in with my therapist and possibly adjust my medication so I can manage this better."

There should be no difference. But because of the stigma, there's still work to be done. As leaders, we have to create an environment where our teams trust us enough to tell the truth about what they're going through—without fear of judgment, shame, or repercussions.

The first thing I believe is essential to establish in your culture is that mental health is a priority. Students in beauty school learn all the basic technical skills needed to perform services. They may even be taught the correct body positioning to help protect their hands, shoulders, and back from strain. But I would be willing to bet that, in most cases, they have not been taught how to properly take care of their mental health. That's where we, as leaders, need to step in and fill the gaps.

Recently, I had a conversation with one of my stylists, and I asked her what had been the most surprising part of her career—something she hadn't expected. She didn't even hesitate before answering.

"I had no idea how emotionally exhausting it would be to work behind the chair with guests all day."

That response didn't surprise me at all.

According to a recent *Modern Salon* article, one in three Americans considers their stylist to be like a therapist. That means our team members are absorbing a lot of emotional baggage—both good and bad—every single day. If they haven't learned how to process that weight correctly, it can build up and become overwhelming.

This is why it's so important to teach them about self-care and help them create their own self-care toolkits—strategies to give their brains a break and protect them from burnout.

Many people assume that burnout comes from the physical demands of the job—and yes, that's part of it. But I would argue that the emotional toll of this work is just as significant, if not more so.

For employees to feel safe talking about mental health, they need to know that it's not just a personal concern—it's a company-wide priority. And that message must come from the top. One of the simplest ways to introduce this in your salon is to include a short conversation about mental health in your next team meeting. It doesn't have to be a big production—just a simple, intentional moment to let them know that their well-being matters.

For me, I chose to lead by being extremely vulnerable and sharing my own experiences with mental health. That level of openness won't be right for every leader, and that's okay. What is important is that the message is clear: mental health is valued and supported here. Beyond just talking about it, we also need to provide a clear path for employees to seek help when they need it. Encourage them to come to you directly if they are struggling, or consider designating a wellness champion on your leadership team —someone they can turn to when they need support. The more we normalize these conversations, the more we create an environment where people feel safe, supported, and valued—not just as employees, but as human beings.

Creating a culture where mental health is prioritized doesn't happen overnight. It requires consistent effort, open conversations, and leading by example. One of the biggest mistakes leaders make is assuming that if their employees needed help, they would ask for it. But the reality is, most people won't—especially in a work environment. They may fear being seen as weak, worry about job security, or simply not know how to bring it up. That's why it's so important to normalize the conversation before someone is in crisis.

I started doing this by integrating small mental health check-ins into our team meetings. Sometimes, it's as simple as asking, *"How's everyone doing? Like, really doing?"* Other times, I might bring up a short topic—something about managing stress, handling overwhelm, or setting boundaries with clients. These moments may seem small, but over time, they help build trust.

I also make it clear that mental health days are just as valid as sick days. If someone calls in saying they have the flu, no one questions it. But if they're having a severe anxiety attack and can't function, why should that be any different? I encourage my team to communicate when they need a break, and I back it up by actually supporting them when they do.

At the same time, I set expectations around self-care. Burnout is real in our industry, and I don't want my stylists waiting until they hit a breaking point before they do something about it. We talk about strategies they can implement—whether it's taking breaks between clients, learning how to leave work at work, setting healthy boundaries, or seeking therapy when needed.

When I first started opening up about my own mental health journey, I wasn't sure how my team would respond. Would they think I was weak? Would they be uncomfortable? Would they take me less seriously as a leader?

Instead, something completely unexpected happened.

One by one, team members started coming to me privately, sharing their own struggles. Some told me about their anxiety. Others opened up about depression, grief, trauma, or medication struggles. Some had never talked about these things with anyone before. And because I had created the space for it, they finally felt safe enough to ask for support.

That was when I knew—this is the kind of leadership that actually matters. It's not just about revenue numbers, social media followers, or how many clients we can squeeze into a day. It's about the people. Because at the end of the day, the success of any business comes down to the well-being of the people who run it. If they are burned out, exhausted, or mentally struggling, the business will struggle too. But if they feel supported, valued, and empowered to take care of themselves, they will thrive—and when they thrive, the business thrives with them.

This is what leadership looks like.

And this is the kind of leader I choose to be.

Determining what benefits you can offer to support mental health is a key step in fostering a workplace culture that prioritizes well-being. Maybe it's adding extra personal days to their allotted time off, offering sick days specifically for mental health, or, in my case, providing an Ally Health benefit that gives each team member access to telehealth services and ten free therapy sessions per year at a very low cost per employee. You might also consider offering a short-term disability policy so that if an employee ever needs extended time off for mental health reasons, they can take it while still receiving a portion of their income.

Beyond direct healthcare support, you can also negotiate discounted memberships with local gyms or yoga studios, or provide access to meditation apps as part of their benefits package. When meeting with employees to set professional goals and map out their career growth, take time to create a self-care plan alongside it—one that helps them strengthen their mental health and prevent burnout.

The old-school mentality in the beauty industry—where stylists were expected to work excessive hours, double-book clients, skip lunch breaks, and sacrifice evenings and weekends—is no longer sustainable. The sooner we implement a more balanced approach to scheduling, the more likely we are to retain talented employees and earn their trust, showing them that we care about their well-being and their paycheck.

As leaders, it's also crucial that we educate ourselves on the warning signs of mental health struggles in our employees. The symptoms of burnout, anxiety, and depression can often look identical to poor performance—low energy, frequent absences, disengagement, or a lack of motivation. Before jumping to conclusions and assuming an employee doesn't care or isn't trying, ask the right questions.

Now, whenever I notice a dip in performance or an emotional outburst from a team member, I start with a simple question:

"How have you been taking care of yourself lately?"

That one question alone can be incredibly powerful. If your team members know they can safely talk to you about their struggles, they will. Instead of making them feel ashamed or guilty for a medical condition beyond their control, you can become a partner in their healing.

If it turns out that an employee is struggling with their mental health, work together to come up with a plan. They might just need a day off or a temporary schedule change to reset. For more serious situations, they may need a leave of absence to seek professional treatment.

Unfortunately, for employees who have never been diagnosed or treated for mental illness before, the journey to recovery can be a long one. Finding the right provider, getting a diagnosis, and experimenting with medications, therapy, and self-care strategies takes time. Unlike treating a physical illness—where a doctor can run tests and prescribe a proven treatment—mental health care is often a process of trial and error.

However, with the right resources and support, it is entirely possible to thrive, even with a severe mental illness. I know this firsthand.

Not everyone's journey will take as long as mine did, but early detection and quick action can make a significant difference. As business owners and leaders, we may be the only person in our employees' lives who can guide them in the right direction.

That being said, there will be times when an employee tries to use mental health as an excuse for poor performance—even when they are not genuinely struggling. I've dealt with this too. The approach should be the same regardless: poor performance cannot be tolerated long-term, but every employee deserves grace during difficult seasons.

If you've worked with an employee to develop a mental health plan and they still aren't following through—whether that means not seeking help, refusing treatment, or failing to take ownership of their well-being—there may come a point where you have to enforce a leave of absence or, in extreme cases, let them go.

However, I firmly believe that if we create a safe environment for employees to be honest about their mental health, we can retain more staff and support them in a way that allows them to recover instead of walking away. Before assuming an employee simply doesn't care, we need to at least consider that mental health may be playing a role in their performance.

This next part is critical—and arguably the most important piece in creating a mentally healthy workplace.

As leaders, we must take responsibility for the impact we have on our team's mental health. Did you know that a manager can have a greater impact on an employee's mental health than their doctor, therapist, or even their partner? Almost 70% of people report that their manager has more influence on their mental health than any medical professional or loved one. (*Forbes*) That means we have to take ownership of our emotional wake—the energy, stress, and baggage we bring into the workplace each day.

We have to ask ourselves:

- Are we contributing to a toxic work culture?
- Are we creating stress or anxiety for our employees?
- Are we setting an example of healthy leadership, or are we unintentionally harming our team's well-being?

If we want to create a positive work experience where employees can thrive emotionally, it starts with us. We have to be willing to evaluate our own mental health and make sure we are modeling the same healthy behaviors we expect from our team. If we are constantly stressed, emotionally unavailable, or dumping our own frustrations onto our staff, it can be incredibly damaging to the culture we are trying to create.

If we aren't prioritizing our own self-care, mental well-being, and personal time, our employees will see that. They won't take us seriously when we tell them to take care of themselves—because we're not even doing it ourselves. Running a business is demanding. It requires strength, resilience, and emotional stability. That's why it is absolutely essential that we commit to our own self-care, set boundaries, and recharge when necessary—so that we can show up as present, supportive, and level-headed leaders for our teams.

At the end of the day, a thriving business is built on healthy, fulfilled, and empowered employees. And as leaders, it's up to us to set the tone for what that looks like.

You may be thinking to yourself, *Why is this my responsibility?* And I get it. As business owners, we already have so much on our plates that adding yet another level of responsibility—caring for our employees' mental health—can feel overwhelming. But the payoff can be enormous.

When people have positive mental health, 63% say they are committed to their work, and 80% say they feel energized (*Forbes*). I don't know about you, but those are exactly the kind of people I want to work with.

You may also be thinking, *Nobody on my staff seems to be struggling with mental health challenges.* But according to the American Association for Suicide Prevention, one in five adults experiences mental illness every year. That means, statistically speaking, several of your employees are likely living with or working through a mental health challenge right now—whether you realize it or not.

Unless, of course, you've already created an environment where they feel safe enough to talk about it. If that's the case, you're already ahead of the game. You should be proud of the leadership you're providing.

But for those who haven't yet taken this step, consider this your nudge.

Don't know where to start? Let's chat. I've paid attention and have accepted my calling. I've taken something horrible that happened TO me and I now know it happened FOR me. I'm on a mission to shatter the stigma and do everything in my power to spread awareness and be the light that someone out there just may be depending on. Let's do this. Let's just start talking more about it. What do you say?

Laura's Self-Care Toolkit

If you don't already have a self-care routine, start one now. It's not a matter of IF you'll need it —it's a matter of WHEN.

My self-care routine includes prioritizing:

- Medication
- Supplements
- Regular health screenings/medication checks
- 8-9 hours of restful sleep nightly
- Drinking 100 oz of water each day
- Limited alcohol (almost never)
- Limited Diet Coke (one per week)
- Eating whole foods
- Exercise 3-5 times per week
- Walks
- Regular massages or Myofascial Release treatments
- Pickleball (it's not just for old people anymore)
- Regular hangouts with my friends—laughing until we cry
- "Estrofest" (my annual girl's trip to FL w/college besties)
- Only the softest pajamas to sleep in
- High thread count sheets
- Candles with my favorite aromas

Laura's Self-Care Toolkit

- Fresh flowers on my desk
- Grocery delivery
- Practicing gratitude
- Finding joy in the little things
- Meditation
- Planning my downtime—resting with the same intensity as I climb
- Binge-watching reality TV shows
- Saying NO more often
- Developing JOMO—joy of missing out

Resources

NAMI.
NAMI. (2024). *Mental Health Conditions | NAMI: National Alliance on Mental Illness.* Www.nami.org. https://www.nami.org/About-Mental-Illness/Mental-Health-Conditions/

Ketamine.
Grinspoon, P. (2024, February 15). *Ketamine for treatment-resistant depression: When and Where Is It safe?* Harvard Health. https://www.health.harvard.edu/blog/ketamine-for-treatment-resistant-depression-when-and-where-is-it-safe-202208092797

Wikipedia Contributors. (2018, December 2). *Ketamine.* Wikipedia; Wikimedia Foundation. https://en.wikipedia.org/wiki/Ketamine

Electroconvulsive Therapy, ECT.
Mayo Clinic. (2018). *Electroconvulsive therapy (ECT).* Mayoclinic.org. https://www.mayoclinic.org/tests-procedures/electroconvulsive-therapy/about/pac-20393894

Transcranial Magnetic Stimulation, TMS.
Mayo Clinic. (2018, November 27). *Transcranial Magnetic Stimulation.* Mayoclinic.org. https://www.mayoclinic.org/tests-procedures/transcranial-magnetic-stimulation/about/pac-20384625

GeneSight Testing.
FAQs | GeneSight. (2023). GeneSight. https://genesight.com/clinician-faq/

Vitamin D and mental health.
Guzek, D., Kołota, A., Lachowicz, K., Skolmowska, D., Stachoń, M., & Głąbska, D. (2021). Association between Vitamin D Supplementation and Mental Health in Healthy Adults: A Systematic Review. *Journal of Clinical Medicine, 10*(21), 5156. https://doi.org/10.3390/jcm10215156

Gut-brain connection.
Robertson, R. (2023, July 31). *The gut-brain connection: How it works and the role of nutrition.* Healthline. https://www.healthline.com/nutrition/gut-brain-connection

MTHFR gene.
Zhang, Y.-X., Yang, L.-P., Gai, C., Cheng, C.-C., Guo, Z., Sun, H.-M., & Hu, D. (2022). Association between variants of MTHFR genes and psychiatric disorders: A

meta-analysis. *Frontiers in Psychiatry, 13.* https://doi.org/10.3389/fpsyt.2022.976428

Alive AF.

Alive AF: One Mom's Journey To Becoming Alcohol Free by Samantha Perkins (2020)

Berberine.

Tang, Y., Su, H., Nie, K., Wang, H., Gao, Y., Chen, S., Lu, F., & Dong, H. (2024). Berberine exerts antidepressant effects in vivo and in vitro through the PI3K/AKT/CREB/BDNF signaling pathway. *Biomedicine & Pharmacotherapy, 170,* 116012–116012. https://doi.org/10.1016/j.biopha.2023.116012

Modern Salon:

Staff, M. (2023, April 24). *1 in 3 Americans View Their Stylist as a Therapist.* Modernsalon.com; Modern Salon. https://www.modernsalon.com/1086840/1-in-3-americans-view-their-stylist-as-a-therapist

NAMI.

National Alliance on Mental Illness. (2023, April). *Mental health by the numbers.* National Alliance on Mental Illness. https://www.nami.org/about-mental-illness/mental-health-by-the-numbers/

Forbes.

Brower, T. (2023, January 29). *Managers Have Major Impact On Mental Health: How To Lead For Wellbeing.* Forbes. https://www.forbes.com/sites/tracybrower/2023/01/29/managers-have-major-impact-on-mental-health-how-to-lead-for-wellbeing/

Acknowledgments

To my children, Julia & Shelby—you are mine and your Dad's greatest accomplishments. You are beautiful, independent young women that I am so proud of and love with all my heart.

To my parents, Rich & Nan—thank you for providing a safe, loving and encouraging family for me to grow up in. I got the best parts of both of you and the gift of a solid foundation on which I've been able to build on and create an amazing life for myself. Thank you for coming back together to save me when I needed you most!

To my sister, Erin—thank you for the time you spent with me, taking me to treatments and making sure I was safe. Your love and friendship means the world to me and I'm so glad we're back to laughing at our own jokes together.

To my manager at Pure, Jennifer—you will never truly know how much I appreciate the sacrifices you've made for me, for stepping up when I couldn't and for the unwavering support you've given to me, our team and the incredible success we've built together. You are one in a million.

To my team at Pure Salon Spa—thank you for believing in me and our team even when I was away, for all of the things you did and took care of that I never knew about, I appreciate all of it.

To my Bad Ass Aveda Owners KY group—I would not have lasted long in this industry without our sisterhood! You guys are the real deal and have carried me through some incredibly difficult seasons over the years—I haven't figured out yet if we're stupid or just crazy for staying in it this long. *Bad ass* doesn't begin to cover it!

To my friend, Samantha Perkins—thank you for inspiring me to write this story. It is through witnessing your courage, I found mine. You are my ambassador of QUAN!

To Amy Meredith, my writing and accountability partner. Thank you for your commitment to meet weekly to write and encourage each other when we got stuck. Those Tuesdays for 90 mins added up over time and led me to publish a memoir! Your friendship is a gift!

To my editor, Becky—thank you for pushing me to see the opportunities for this memoir through a bigger lens. Working on this project together has been a highlight in my journey and I can't imagine having done it with anyone but you.

To my friend, Holly—thank you for holding space for me while I cried and tried to explain the darkness that had become my new normal. Your compassion and understanding that day made me feel seen and gave me hope.

To my friend, Melinda—thank you for your friendship, support and connection over mummified pups. Your kindred spirit was a lifeline to me as I navigated life as a military spouse and I will never forget the fun we've had together.

To my EstroFest Crew—you are the absolute best friends a girl could ever ask for. Hands down, your friendships are among the greatest gifts I've been given in this life. In my heart, you will always remain Honorable, Beautiful and Highest.

To Dr. Timothy Burke—thank you for spending more than two hours with my husband and I at the first appointment and taking me on as a patient even though you were only months from retirement. I am so grateful you cared enough at a time I needed it most. Your commitment to providing me the best care is the reason I'm alive and thriving.

To Dr. Ronald Spears—thank you for taking over my treatments after Dr. Burke retired and assisting me on the path to thriving again. Please don't take this the wrong way but I hope to never need to see you again as a patient!

To The Brook Hospital—thank you for providing ECT services to the Louisville community. Your staff does amazing, important work and the ECT crew handled my care with compassion and dignity.

To Danielle & The Couch Mental Health Care—thank you for finding the right combination of medications to keep me out of the deep dark hole I found myself in. Thank you for asking the questions that had never been asked before and for teaching me to take a holistic approach to my healing. Your compassion and connection came just in time.

To all of you near and far who kept me in your thoughts and prayers while I was in the dark, THANK YOU!

To those of you who are suffering in silence, I see you and I know you are tired! You are worthy of thriving and there is a solution for you too. Keep reaching out and trying the next thing. It's not your fault. Keep advocating for yourself until you find the light.

About the Author

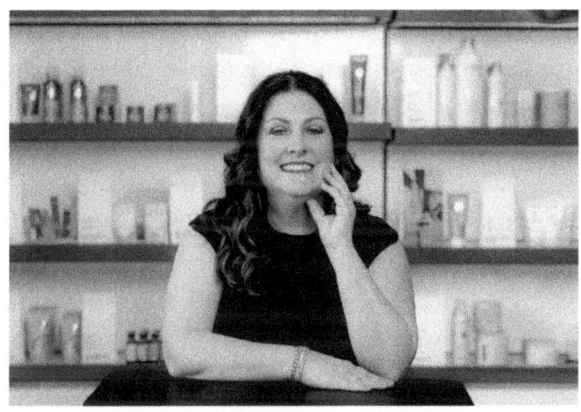

Laura Watkins is the owner of Pure Salon Spa, an Aveda salon and spa recognized among the Top 200 salons in North America. A respected voice in the beauty industry, Laura also serves as a "Purefessor" with the Aveda Business College, where she shares her expertise in business development and leadership with salon owners across the country. She holds a bachelor's degree in Marketing and an MBA from the University of Louisville, as well as a professional cosmetology license. Laura lives in Louisville, Kentucky, with her husband, Mike. Together, they have two daughters, Julia and Shelby.

After battling treatment-resistant major depressive disorder that nearly claimed her life, Laura has become a passionate advocate for mental health awareness. She serves on the board of directors for Mental Health Lou, a nonprofit working to ensure that mental wellness remains at the center of community conversations. Through this work and her personal story, Laura is helping to break the stigma surrounding mental illness and create safer spaces for honest dialogue and support.

With *Something Feels Off*, Laura hopes to use her platform to educate others about the power of self-care as a form of preventative care—especially within high-pressure service industries like beauty and wellness. She is committed to training salon owners and industry leaders to recognize the signs of mental health challenges, foster supportive workplace cultures, and integrate mental wellness into the fabric of how salons operate. Her mission is clear: to spark a movement in which compassion, transparency, and self-care are just as essential as creativity and client service.

By sharing her journey, Laura offers hope to those who feel lost in their own struggles. She reminds us all that our mental health should be a priority along with physical health and healing is not only possible—it can become a powerful catalyst for change.

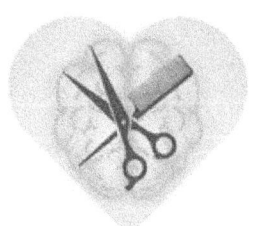

Invite Laura to speak at your event or find out more about how to bring her work to life in your organization.

Email her at laura@puresalon-spa.com
Follow her on Instagram @mental_girl502
Visit her website www.mentalgirl502.com

www.ingramcontent.com/pod-product-compliance
Lightning Source LLC
Chambersburg PA
CBHW032112040426
42337CB00040B/227